Men's Health

For Churchill Livingstone

Senior Commissioning Editor: Alex Mathieson
Project Development Editor: Mairi McCubbin
Design Direction: Judith Wright

Men's Health
An Introduction for Nurses and Health Professionals

Edited by

Tony Harrison BA RN RSCN RNT
Nurse Teacher, University of Manchester, School of Nursing, Midwifery and Health Visiting, Manchester, UK

Karen Dignan Msc ADM FP Cert MTD CertEd RN RM
Midwife Teacher, University of Manchester, School of Nursing, Midwifery and Health Visiting, Manchester, UK

Foreword by

Steve Jamieson MSc BSc(Hons) RMN RGN DipCPN
Adviser in Men's Health and Sexual Health, The Royal College of Nursing, London, UK

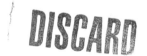
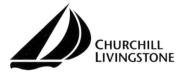

CHURCHILL
LIVINGSTONE

EDINBURGH LONDON NEW YORK PHILADELPHIA SYDNEY TORONTO 1999

CHURCHILL LIVINGSTONE
An imprint of Harcourt Brace and Company Limited

© Harcourt Brace and Company Limited 1999

⚓ is a registered trade mark of Harcourt Brace and Company Limited 1999

First published 1999

ISBN 0 443 059195

British Library Cataloguing in Publication Data
A catalogue record for this book is available from the British Library.

Library of Congress Cataloging in Publication Data
A catalog record for this book is available from the Library of Congress.

Note
Medical knowledge is constantly changing. As new information becomes available, changes in treatment, procedures, equipment and the use of drugs become necessary. The editors, contributors and the publishers have, as far as it is possible, taken care to ensure that the information given in this text is accurate and up to date. However, readers are strongly advised to confirm that the information, especially with regard to drug usage, complies with latest legislation and standards of practice.

The
publisher's
policy is to use
**paper manufactured
from sustainable forests**

Printed in China
NPCC/01

Contents

Contributors

Karen Dignan MSc ADM FP Cert MTD CertEd RN RM
Midwifery Teacher, University of Manchester, School of Nursing, Midwifery and Health Visiting, Manchester, UK

Christine M. Furber MSc BSc RN RM ADM CertEd MTD
Midwifery Teacher, University of Manchester, School of Nursing, Midwifery and Health Visiting, Manchester, UK

Tony Harrison BA RN RSCN RNT
Nurse Teacher, University of Manchester, School of Nursing, Midwifery and Health Visiting, Manchester, UK

Kevin Mullarkey MA(Couns) BSc(Hons) CPNCert RNT RMN RGN
Nurse Teacher, University of Manchester, School of Nursing, Midwifery and Health Visiting, Manchester, UK

Judith Ormrod MSc BSc BEd DipCouns Dpn RNT RN
University of Manchester, School of Nursing, Midwifery and Health Visiting, Manchester, UK

Elizabeth H. E. Pease FRCOG FRCS(Ed)
Consultant in Reproductive Medicine, Department of Reproductive Medicine, St Mary's Hospital, Manchester, UK

John F. Playle MSc BSc(Hons) DipCouns RN CPNCert RNT
Senior Lecturer in Health and Social Care, School of Human and Health Sciences, University of Huddersfield, Huddersfield, UK

Karen Price
Stepping Hill Hospital, Stockport, UK

Catherine Rhodes MSc RGN RNT DipN(Lond) CertCouns
Counselling Services Coordinator, University of Manchester, School of Nursing, Midwifery and Health Visiting, Manchester, UK

Howard Shilton MSc MA BA RGN DipN(Lond)
Lecturer in Nursing, University of Manchester, School of Nursing, Midwifery and Health Visiting, Manchester, UK

Paul Shilton AIBMS BSc(Hons)
Biomedical Scientist, Department of Pathology, North Manchester Healthcare NHS Trust, Manchester, UK

Carole A. Webb DipMid RM RGN
Midwifery Sister, Marron Maternity Unit, Royal Oldham Hospital, Oldham, UK

Foreword

The issue of 'men's health' in its own right has attracted considerable interest in recent years. During the last period of Conservative government the role of the NHS shifted from one of treating sickness to that of promoting health, placing emphasis on the individual's capacity to change his or her own behaviour. The current Labour government aims to take this a stage further. The recent Green Paper on public health, *Our Healthier Nation*, sets out the case for 'concerted action to tackle not just the causes of the disease but the causes of the causes'.

This new agenda intends to encourage normal healthy lifestyles for the majority of people. More men than women are born every year and yet they have a shorter lifespan, fewer men consult their doctors, and men have higher rates of admission to hospital, a widely accepted indicator of serious health problems. Areas of major concern in men's health are coronary heart disease, testicular and prostate cancers, sexual health, accidents at work and mental health, especially suicide. Men and women have a different perception of their health. Men stress being fit, strong and energetic while women stress not being ill and never seeing a doctor.

The Green Paper sets out ways to tackle root causes of ill health and concentrates on four areas: heart disease, cancers, accidents at work and mental health. It is important to note that we are not developing health services and initiatives for men just because there are similar services available for women. Thus, one argument is that there should be screening for prostate cancer simply because there is a screening programme for breast cancer. Others have stated that 'women have had their health needs met for the last 20 years and now it's men's turn to fight back'.

Broadening the context in which we think about men's health also exposes the lack of existing research data on men. This is a difficult issue that needs to be addressed quickly. It will be essential to carry out appropriate research and develop comprehensive data bases and suitable evaluation methods to highlight examples of good practice. All involved in men's health need to be prepared to function effectively in a constantly changing health service and respond to the needs of society. What is meant by men's health will inevitably expand further with the new definition of public health, bringing to the fore, social, economic and environmental issues.

It is a privilege to write this foreword as the men's health adviser and coordinator of the Men's Health Forum (MHF). The MHF was established in 1994 as a national, independent and representative body. The forum aims to provide a platform for interested organizations and industries to discuss, disseminate and promote ideas on men's health and to contribute to the development of good practice.

This book will prove to be an invaluable resource, as a research-orientated source of knowledge that addresses and influences both practice and a greater awareness of the broader issues of men's health.

1999   Steve Jamieson

Preface

Only comparatively recently has men's health achieved status as an entity in its own right. The reasons for this are somewhat complex. It would be simplistic to suggest that men's health has become an issue because in some quantifiable way the state of the health of men in the UK has decreased markedly in recent years. We certainly can identify trends in ill health distinct to the male gender, which need to be addressed by the health care system, but relegating men's health to disease association alone would be a retrograde step in our understanding of the concept of health as a whole.

Arguably, the women's health movement has identified the efficacy of looking not only at the disease process specific to gender, but also at the characteristics and experiences of that gender which underlie ill health for that sex. Such a holistic approach to health is central to the philosophies of care espoused by most groups of health care professionals.

The definition of what constitutes women's health generically continues to evolve and its evolution predates any such definition for men's health by decades; but the process has commenced. This text seeks to contribute to the debate rather than to complete it. We would argue that now is the time for such a debate. Health care professionals should capitalize on the current media interest in 'men's health', expanding what might be seen as a predominantly white, middle-class preoccupation with physique and prowess into a true health agenda, one which seeks to take the possibly trite and make of it a proactive exploration of gender-based health in all its facets.

The contributors to this text are professionals in health care and represent both genders. A deviation from the philosophies of some strands of the women's health movement in our case must be that issues around gender-related health can be explored and indeed learned by any professional regardless of gender. Gender-specific health care in the UK is not a reality if the gender in question is that of the professional carer. Most such professionals in health and social care are women, who have amassed expertise and skill in exploring and meeting the health care needs of men because that is their professional role. To negate or underplay this is to deny the ability of professionals to intervene effectively with a range of groups with whom they do not necessarily share distinct characteristics. Sharing characteristics makes empathy more possible, but professional application and learning can, we believe, achieve the same end, particularly if it is based on learning from the clients themselves. In this, perhaps, the men's health debate has something to contribute to the women's health movement.

The University of Manchester School of Nursing, Midwifery and Health Visiting recently received approval to develop the ENB A89, a course designed to explore issues of men's health and their efficacious application to practice. In researching literature for this course, it became evident that literature on men's health fell into two distinct categories: the popularist texts largely written for the public, which tend to focus on virility, physique, hair loss and self-esteem; and the professional, pertinent research-based pieces scattered through the 'ologies'. Texts which address men's health as a primary focus were, however, rare, startlingly so when compared with similar texts on women's health. This being the case, we decided to produce our own.

This text is principally a reference text and sections may be read as distinct entities or, more valuably, the text may be taken as a whole in order for the reader to gain a clear view of this complex subject.

Specialization in health care has focused on the disease or its process – cardiology, urology, intensive care, etc. Women's health has been a notable departure from this. We believe that the uncounted number of carers whose specialities are more generic, such as community, male medicine and male surgery, have had their actual specialism – men's health – overlooked. Their skills and experience in dealing with the health of a specific gender (frequently and importantly not their own gender in most cases) warrant both exploration and validation.

We hope that you enjoy the text and would welcome feedback via the editors. Even more, we hope that this text helps to encourage interest and debate in this relatively new subject, wherever that debate may lead.

Manchester, 1999

Karen Dignan
Tony Harrison

1

Men's health: the background

Carole Ann Webb

Introduction
Past development of services
What is available now
The development of the well man
   clinic
Consultation times
Male or female staff?
Doctors or nurses?
Private or public sector?
Clinic venue

Common health issues
Coronary heart disease
Smoking
Alcohol
Stress
Cancer
Osteoporosis
Sexual health
Diet
The future of men's health

INTRODUCTION

The whole area of men's health is greatly undervalued, be it by men themselves or by providers of health care, and yet men's life expectancy is more than 5 years less than women's (Calman 1992). Why this is so is not clearly understood and there may be several issues involved, but it is clear that the problem needs addressing. This can be done either by the initiative of the men who use health care or by the staff who provide this care.

The first health visitors to set up a well man clinic in Glasgow suggested that 'The family car probably receives more care and maintenance than the average adult man'. It may be a generalization, but it tends to be women who initiate better health care for men. For instance, it is mothers and wives who most often do the cooking, so a healthy diet in this case would depend upon the knowledge and cooking skills of the woman involved. Women can play a big part in encouraging men to attend the doctor either for treatment when they are ill or for screening. Perhaps due to their maternal role or due to the history of women's health screening where women had to lobby for certain services, they may feel that if men cannot or will not seek out better services, then they will have to encourage them to do it.

The media could play a bigger role in trying to improve men's health. Many medical programmes are shown on television but very few are aimed specifically at men. Newspapers carry articles and medical sections with answers to readers' questions given by doctors, but these still largely cover women's health or more general issues. Men's journals are very few and far between and most only cover topics such as sport or car and home maintenance and any that are connected with health are usually geared towards body building or physical attractiveness rather than the maintenance of good health. With the increased interest in computers and the Internet, it would be useful to have a website for both male and female health, as many men enjoy technology and may seek out information specific to them. The health service itself could also increase its role in improving men's health from the government down to individual health care trusts.

Government funding is available for specific health initiatives such as the advertising campaigns relating to AIDS and smoking. These are carried out by the Health Education Authority (HEA) which is funded partly by the Department of Health, by sales of its publications and by the World Health Organization. It could be more advantageous for the HEA to initiate a men's health campaign as better funding may be available using this source rather than depending on NHS trusts which have several priorities. This does not exclude trusts from taking responsibility for men's health issues; in fact, if they do not invest in the health of the men in their locality, then the cost of care when men become ill will fall on the trust.

The cost of medical care is greater than the cost of health education, so money spent on prevention would seem prudent. However, the results are not necessarily seen for many years so this may lead to a reluctance on the part of local trust managers to become involved in men's health education as they would be paying for a service of which their successors would reap the benefits. It is largely the local Family Health Services Authority (FHSA) who funds men's health clinics via GPs. The FHSA cannot insist that a GP sets up a well man clinic, it only pays for its funding, so the GP has to initiate the setting up of such a clinic. If enough men can be encouraged to attend, this can lead to quite a sizeable monetary incentive for the practice.

From an early age, children learn the hidden agenda provided by adults; for instance, if a little girl falls down and is hurt she can expect to be picked up and cuddled, almost rewarded for the injury, and she is made to feel better. Little boys, on the other hand, can expect to be picked up and told not to cry but to be a 'brave little boy'. Sabo & Gordon (1995) identified that sex role theorists and feminist theorists agreed that the social construction of masculinity produces a negative impact on men's health. The hidden message here is that males are almost expected to put up with discomfort and not to seek attention or assistance. If this message continues to be reinforced then, as an adult, it may be very difficult for a man to overcome it. A reversal of these attitudes is required to ensure the health of future generations. The difficulty lies in finding an effective, long-lasting method of changing these deeply entrenched attitudes.

PAST DEVELOPMENT OF SERVICES

When we think of women's health issues, there are many aspects that can be included. Indeed, from the menarche to the menopause and beyond, women have access to health care screening that men should feel envious of. There are family planning clinics, antenatal clinics, triannual cervical screening programmes and mammography, to name but a few. The improvement in women's health care and screening services was largely due to women demanding these services themselves (Deans 1988). They grew from the women's movements of the 1960s along with demands for equal pay and conditions in the workplace and men missed their opportunity to demand their rights to equal health care and health screening. It was also during this time that one of the few screening services for men was ending – the medical for National Service. Although not everyone was called up for service, a large proportion of the adult male population would have had the benefit of the medical. Although it was never meant as a means of educating men into better health by trying to reduce habits such as smoking or excessive alcohol consumption, it would have detected any medical risk factors.

The reasons why women felt that they needed better services but men continued to be complacent about their health are unknown.

WHAT IS AVAILABLE NOW

So what about current screening services for men? Apart from medical examinations through private screening or when seeking new employment, there is very little provision for men's health care and men seem to be let down very badly.

With the advent of internal marketing, detailed in the Government White Paper *Working for patients* (1989), some GPs set up well man clinics. These clinics attract funding from the local FHSA and initially, to qualify for funding, a clinic had to have at least 10 men attending in one session but this was difficult for some practices to achieve. The FHSAs relented and began to allow funding for every 10 men who attended whenever the appointments occurred. By changing this rule, more GPs were able to continue to offer a well man clinic, so here at least was a positive step towards men's future health.

The protocols are agreed by each individual practice, usually between the GP and the practice nurse, and so the services offered will differ from practice to practice. The usual inclusions are details of family history and own past medical history, blood pressure measurement, weight and height (in order to calculate the body mass index), age and urinalysis. For men with a family history of coronary heart disease (CHD), cholesterol estimation may be carried out and, finally, information on testicular self-examination may be given. There are no guidelines as to how often a well man check should be carried out.

THE DEVELOPMENT OF THE WELL MAN CLINIC

The first well man clinic was set up in the early part of the 1980s and was started by health care professionals, unlike women's screening services which were largely consumer led (Sadler 1985). The intention was not to develop a medical model whereby disease was identified and then referred to a medical practitioner but to establish a means of identifying lifestyle risk factors that could later develop into a medical problem. Once identified, these risks could be discussed with the client and workable steps decided upon to improve their lifestyle, with the resultant reduction in future ill health. These clinics differed little from the clinics of today, with the emphasis being placed on CHD screening.

Initially, health visitors began setting up these well man clinics and they included them in their weekly schedule rather than running them in addition to it. Health visitors felt well placed to undertake this role as their training centres around health promotion rather than screening for illness. The venue of the clinic varied from place to place, some in the local health centre, others in the GP's practice. As the clinics began to evolve, many health authorities began to feel they could no longer support the cost of them via the health visiting service. With the effects not being seen immediately, they felt the cost was unjustifiable.

Following the Government White Paper *Working for patients* (1989) and with the new GP Contract, more well man clinics were set up by GPs, especially when they were allowed to hold their own budgets from April 1990. The GP Contract was meant to make health promotion and disease prevention part of the work of all GPs. These health promotion clinics were set up in surgeries and clinics at the local practice. More practice nurses were employed and funding was available for them to obtain education in this field, although it was not necessary to hold the Practice Nurse Certificate to obtain employment in this area. This meant that some nurses who had never had experience of screening or health education became responsible for it. Now that nurses are being made more responsible for their continuing education due to Post Registration Education and Practice (PREP) (UKCC 1997), this should encourage a higher standard of care. Nurses are required to maintain knowledge and competence in their field of nursing practice. As many clinics run by the practice nurse are for women, they require new skills such as being able to undertake a cervical smear. Study days may be used to increase awareness of women's health but there is no guarantee that men's health matters will be studied.

There is very little written about men's health clinics which may, in part, be due to the relatively low profile these clinics have. No new ideas seem to have been put forward on either the running or the content of these clinics and the emphasis remains on CHD screening and the reduction/discontinuation of habits such as smoking and alcohol consumption. Although these are causes of morbidity/mortality in men, there are many other issues which need to be addressed. A Royal College of Physicians report on the prevention of CHD emphasized concentrating on this group to reduce the risk factors (Wrench & Irvine 1984).

Since the first clinics were set up in Sussex in 1981 and Castlemilk, Glasgow, in 1984, little has changed in the way men are encouraged to attend well man clinics. Then, men were actively recruited by invitation and in most of the GP clinics, this is still the main method used today. Some GP practices send letters of invitation to men within a certain age group to attend for a health check and this may be backed up by a further letter if there is no response to the first one. Other practices rely on poster advertising within the surgery, giving details of the availability of men's clinics and some of the services offered, such as blood pressure estimation. This would only capture the attention of men who are already attending the GP, so other men may miss the opportunity of having a health check. This group may contain the men who are in greatest need of health advice.

The GP Contract of 1990 stated that health promotion and disease prevention, including the provision of advice through regular check-ups and screening, should be part of the work of all general practitioners. Some GPs took this literally and chose to undertake the screening themselves, opportunistically, within the consultation time. Others employed practice nurses to do this, having then been granted more funds to employ practice staff. This may have seemed a costly exercise initially, to employ a qualified nurse to undertake health promotion where the benefits may not be seen for years, if ever. With the introduction of GP fundholding in April 1991, the benefits of employing a nurse were easier to see. The nurse could undertake the running of asthma clinics, diabetic clinics and other such clinics that the GPs were then having to purchase as a service from the local trust hospitals. The FHSA would fund the practice for these clinics so the more clinics a practice had, the wealthier it would become, with more money available for further initiatives.

CONSULTATION TIMES

As previously mentioned, some doctors tried to incorporate health promotion into the medical consultation but how effective could this be, given the amount of time available and the lack of planning for each client? How responsive would the client be if they had gone to see the doctor with other worries or physical illness? It is interesting to note that one research paper investigated whether extending the length of the consultation time from 7.5 min to 10 min per patient would increase health promotion in general practice (Wilson et al 1992). They concluded that consultation times should be increased to 10 min, as part of that time would have to be spent on the problem the patient had attended for, leaving very little time available for health promotion.

When the first clinics were set up in the 1980s the nurses usually allowed 30 min for a consultation and often these were found to overrun. It is surely better to have a longer consultation time to allow for a detailed examination of lifestyle and physical statistics (height, weight, etc.) and for information to be given on how and why changes can be made and the advantages of doing so. A follow-up appointment can also be given to see how changes are being made or, if not, whether goals need to be altered. It should be borne in mind, though, that a busy GP may be reluctant to initiate a follow-up appointment.

The fact that doctors see a 10 min consultation as suitable for a full health care screening perhaps indicates that some of them see men's health as low priority. Further studies could be initiated to find the ideal length for a consultation. Perhaps the duration of a consultation is of greater importance to men as they may be anxious if it is lengthy, wondering what will happen within the allotted half hour, but if men are given the chance to control the length of the consultation, then perhaps more men would be encouraged to come forward for health assessment.

MALE OR FEMALE STAFF?

One of the concerns men may have could be with regard to who would run the clinic. At one clinic, the men were asked about their preference for male or female staff and although 76% had no preference, the remainder indicated they would prefer a male member of staff (Brown & Lunt 1992). They may prefer a male if intimate details are to be given or if a physical examination is to take place as they may feel a man can empathize with their needs and not worry about the language they use to describe things. Some may prefer a female who they may see as being more sympathetic and less likely to make them feel awkward if they become embarrassed about a problem.

Gender may perhaps have less significance than the role of the professional and if there is a choice between a female GP and a male practice nurse, this may confuse the client even further. Is the GP seen as having better health promotion skills (due to the nature of their training and therefore more knowledge) regardless of gender or would the nurse be seen as having more time and counselling skills than the doctor, whether male or female? Perhaps only a few men see the issue of gender as the reason why they do not seek health promotion but maybe the doctors and nurses involved in GP health clinics see gender or qualifications as more of a problem.

DOCTORS OR NURSES?

Although it may seem beneficial to have the practice nurse running the health promotion clinics, some GPs are unwilling to give up this role as they believe they are more effective at giving advice and getting clients to change lifestyle habits, e.g. smoking. In a survey in Oxfordshire in 1991, it was found that only 30.2% of the doctors surveyed referred clients to the practice nurse and that was for weight loss and dietary advice (Coulter & Schofield 1991). No reasons were given as to why the doctors did not refer clients more often to the practice nurse or why only weight was used as the basis for a referral.

The health promotion conducted by GPs lays heavy emphasis on CHD and hypertension and although these are the highest causes of premature deaths, there are other issues that could be tackled in a well man clinic. Doctors may feel that they do not have the time for other issues or that only these important health problems need to be addressed in surgery time. Ignorance of what the practice nurse is capable of may prevent referral to the nurse by the doctor. Doctors may be the employers of the practice nurses but not all will be aware of the content of nurse training or of what postregistration training has been undertaken by their particular practice nurse. Many practices will fund further certificated courses for nurses but not be aware of the added skills this will mean for the benefit of the practice. Practice nurses are capable of setting up and running asthma clinics, diabetic clinics and others where men can be recruited for a fuller well man check. Once lifestyle problems have been identified, then further follow-up appointments can be made to check on progress or reassess what further measures might be needed to effect a change in lifestyle.

PRIVATE OR PUBLIC SECTOR?

So far, only NHS clinics have been discussed. The private sector also has several well man clinics in operation. These may be in private hospitals, with their services bought either by individuals or by companies for the purpose of screening employees as part of an occupational health package. There are also private clinics which exist purely to provide well man screening. Although these are obviously more expensive to individuals, the services offered differ too. The professional running the clinic will be a doctor with a nurse or a non-medical person assisting. Because the doctor is employed purely in the capacity of a screening agent and not as a diagnostician, there are no other demands on their time and the consultation time can be from 30 min to 1 h but the cost of this is prohibitive. There are relatively few independent well man clinics and the type of man who is likely to take advantage of them would be middle class, perhaps already aware of health issues and who eats a better diet and takes exercise. The fact that GP well man clinics are free could be used to greater advantage in advertising and in promoting their use. If men know that they can have a free check-up and advice which can cost upwards of £100 privately, then they may be more willing to attend – why turn down an offer of something for nothing?

CLINIC VENUE

The venue of the well man clinic may be of greater importance to men than it would be to women. At one recent clinic run in a health centre there were very few attenders, but when the venue was changed to a local pub, the attendance increased and it was thought this was because the clinic was taken to the men (Baker 1996–7). This surely gives mixed messages, in that alcohol consumption is frowned upon but it is acceptable to use a pub to deliver health information. It could be argued, though, that health information at an unhealthy venue is better than no information at all.

COMMON HEALTH ISSUES

Coronary heart disease

Coronary heart disease (CHD) is still the most common cause of premature death in men. The *Health of the Nation* (1992) included a target to reduce CHD in people under 65 by 40% by the year 2000.

The focus of health clinics is to prevent CHD by obtaining a family history of the disease going back at least two generations, by checking on current lifestyle and by trying to discourage smoking, encourage a low-fat diet (which may also involve weight reduction) and encourage more exercise. A blood pressure measurement is taken to give a baseline and to alert the health professional to a raised blood pressure.

A serum cholesterol measurement may be taken but this is of no value unless some counselling service is available. It is pointless to measure the serum cholesterol level if the client would be reluctant to change his lifestyle if it is found to be high and this may cause added stress. Some would say that it is still necessary to find the serum cholesterol level as it may encourage the client to change his lifestyle if he is aware of how high it is. A problem might arise if the level is quite low as not only would there be no improvement in lifestyle but the client may increase his bad habits thinking, wrongly, that if his cholesterol is low with his current lifestyle then he has no need to worry. However, if there is a genuine desire to act upon the findings of a high cholesterol level then it is useful to take a measurement to enable any improvements to be monitored or, if there is no improvement, then referral can be made to the doctor. Baker (1996–7) states that research undertaken in a well man clinic in mid-Wales found that attendance at such a clinic made no difference to the mean cholesterol or blood pressure levels.

Smoking

Smoking and alcohol consumption are not only associated with CHD but they create problems of their own. Although more women are taking up smoking than ever before, men are still the most likely to become smokers and there are more male than female smokers. The problems of smoking are well documented and can be found in more detail elsewhere. In a leaflet published by the HEA, it is stated that 'Around 5000 British people die in road accidents each year, smoking kills more than 20 times as many'. Deaths can be due to lung cancer, chronic bronchitis with emphysema and, of course, CHD. There are also problems of passive smoking which smokers may not consider or may choose to ignore. If there are children in the household then this may be used to encourage men to give up smoking or at least smoke away from the children. They should be given information on the rise of asthma in children and the risks of lung cancer due to passive smoking.

Alcohol

Alcohol can also cause problems other than helping to increase blood pressure. It causes hepatitis (with vitamin deficiency) and cirrhosis, when consumed over a long period. Gastric problems such as gastritis and ulcers can develop and it can lead to cancer of the mouth, throat and oesophagus (HEA 1994). Other problems include alcohol dependency, days lost from work due to the effects of excessive consumption, depression, impotence and accidents at home and work. Deaths due to drink driving have been steadily falling over the past decade but drink driving still accounted for 500 deaths in 1993 and around 100 000 people are prosecuted each year. A loss of licence can lead to a loss of livelihood and an increase in stress. This is another lifestyle risk that needs to be identified in order to maintain not only good physical health but also good mental health.

Stress

Stress is increasing in the male population, one reason for which may be that more men are reporting stress now instead of coping alone. As the unemployment figures rise and more men are out of work or employed on a part-time basis only, few jobs can be seen as jobs for life and this can lead to an increase in stress.

One outcome of the many stressors of modern living is the recently coined phrase 'road rage'. This demonstrates how stress can lead to violent behaviour if it is not dealt with. Men need to become more open about discussing problems and not feel that they might have failed if they cannot cope alone. One study in America (Matthews 1988) suggests that relating to their families more and being more honest about their inner feelings have reduced men's stress and incidence of CHD by about 20%.

Cancer

Testicular cancer is another area of men's health that needs a higher profile. Although still relatively rare, with around 1400 new cases a year in the UK, it is one of the most curable cancers, with 90% of patients making a full recovery (DoH 1995). Men need to be aware of the factors that increase the risk of having testicular cancer, such as an undescended testicle in childhood, but, more importantly, they should be informed of the symptoms and of how to perform testicular self-examination. It is also necessary to act upon any untoward findings. Kelly (1992) emphasizes this, saying that self-diagnosis can lead to a delay in action due to a fear that the diagnosis will be confirmed. There are several leaflets available from various sources, such as companies that manufacture condoms, cancer charities and from local health authorities. As this cancer can affect even teenagers, it is of vital importance that men are educated as early as possible, by teaching self-examination. Deans (1988) points out two advantages here, in that regular self-examination allows early recognition of changes and a reduction in inhibitions about our 'naughty bits', resulting in an ability to talk freely about worries related to them. If genitalia are discussed openly from an early age there is a tendency to be less self-conscious and the appropriate language can be learned.

Coupled with testicular self-examination, there is the opportunity to question men over the age of 50 about any prostatic changes and to teach them what they should be aware of. As many enlarged prostate glands are benign, this should be one of the first things pointed out to allay any anxiety. Any changes in toilet habits should be discussed such as dribbling or difficulty in passing urine, particularly at night. It may be difficult for men to seek help about urinary symptoms but if the subject is broached during a screening visit then it may become easier to discuss the problem. There is a specific blood test which can be done to identify prostatic cancer, the prostate-specific antigen (PSA) test, which, although costly, is of value if there are already symptoms. It is performed as routine in some of the private well man clinics at a cost of about £50. A study carried out at Manchester University concluded that self-examination and screening by professionals did not affect the stage at which tumours were detected (Buetow 1996).

Osteoporosis

Although osteoporosis is considered to be only a problem for women, one in every 12 men is also at risk of developing this disease. This can be due to a lack of testosterone but other causes can be alcohol or tobacco abuse or the use of steroids.

Although steroids are used as a treatment for many conditions and therefore some kind of monitoring should be in place, a growing number of men are abusing these substances. Body builders generally rely on their own ability to increase muscle bulk by using exercise and diet but some athletes are starting to use anabolic steroids to build bigger muscles than they could ever achieve with diet and exercise alone and although these substances are illegal, they remain uncomfortably accessible. Although Klein (1995) highlighted a 1991 US Department of Health report on steroid abuse by 250 000 high school senior males, he still maintains the root cause of this health risk is to be found in the sport of body-building. Whenever there is an athletics meeting, even at international level, steroid abuse is widely reported in the press. This has been the case in recent years even at the Olympic games, where athletes have been disqualified with much publicity. It seems ironic that men who would appear to be informed on health and well-being actually take steps that are detrimental to their long-term health.

Men attending a well man clinic can be given information to prevent the effects of osteoporosis and this is of greater value in younger men. Simply because the disease is known to affect mostly women, we should not ignore the many men who could be at risk from this debilitating and largely controllable problem.

Sexual health

Sexual health is another issue to be considered and this may simply be contraceptive advice or information on other aspects of sexuality. For many years it has been accepted that contraception is the domain of the woman but this should not be so and men should be encouraged to take responsibility for seeking appropriate advice. Problems such as impotence can be due to many simple factors such as alcohol or stress and advice can be given by someone in the well man clinic but if the problem is outside the scope of this professional, they will be able to refer on to the correct agency.

Advice on sexual health is more important than ever with problems such as hepatitis B and human immunodeficiency virus (HIV) which can be sexually transmitted, both having increased as major killers over the last decade or so. Advice on safer sex needs to be available to both straight and gay men and although leaflets are available, if the advice is given by an individual there is then the opportunity to discuss and ask questions. The right language needs to be used when giving this advice, preferably using non-medical terms and, most importantly, a non-judgemental stance. As part of the clinic, hepatitis B vaccine could be recommended or even given to high-risk men. These may be at higher risk not just because of their sexual activities but also because of their occupations such as refuse collectors or hospital porters, who may be at risk of needlestick injuries, as well as ambulance, police and firemen who will come into contact with blood and other body fluids.

Diet

Dietary advice may also be needed by men, either to lose weight or to eat in a more healthy way. Traditionally, men are fed by women, either their mothers or partners, but as men's role in society is changing more men need to cook for themselves and possibly others as more women work in full-time employment and marriages break down, causing more single-parent families. Dietary advice can be included in a health education session but if weight loss is needed, some men may find it embarrassing to enrol in one of the very popular, but predominantly female, slimming clubs. They may not, however, feel as threatened by attending a well man clinic, where advice can be given on a one-to-one basis.

THE FUTURE OF MEN'S HEALTH

In the main, the biggest problem surrounding men's health is their reluctance to take the opportunities to improve their knowledge and lifestyle. It is not statistics on numbers of deaths that men need but ways in which they can improve their own lives.

To overcome these problems, there needs to be a massive change in the way society sees men's health. This should begin at school where boys can learn not only about their bodies, but also about the social aspects of taking responsibility for their own care and demanding equal status with women's health. It is usual in schools for boys and girls to be separated for gym lessons. As gym teachers have had training in human anatomy, it may be useful to expand this to physiology and health which would then make gym lessons an ideal time to teach some basics of health. There would be less embarrassment in single-sex classes for some issues to be covered but whenever possible, it would be of value to have coeducational teaching to further reduce the taboos surrounding men's health and to understand how females deal with health advice. At present, these subjects may be covered in personal and social education classes and although it is usually only sex education that is taught, it does take the form of a discussion rather than a lecture. This is an improvement on the sex education of the past which was taught in science classes and treated as a very clinical subject where feelings and emotions were ignored. The younger boys are when they feel able to talk openly about their bodies and feelings, the less self-conscious they will be when seeking health advice and this will lead to a potentially healthier adulthood.

Once boys have left the education system, they may find it more diffi-cult to access health information. Employers should be encouraged to provide some kind of health screening and though some employers do already provide excellent occupational health facilities, others provide nothing at all. Legislation to remedy this is not necessarily the answer, as some smaller firms would not be able to afford such a service and would either provide a poor service or have to close down their business. Instead, the government could give incentives to firms willing to provide this service. As not all men are in employment, this could mean that some are overlooked when it comes to health screening. One means of preventing this might be to offer a health screen to men on Social Security benefit, which could be offered when men go to make their claim for Job Seeker's Allowance or when they have been in receipt of benefits for longer than a year. Many people who have seen their benefits cut over recent years may be suspicious of this, seeing it as a means of finding them unfit for work, for instance, or seeing how they spend their benefit money. They may give incorrect answers as to alcohol and nicotine consumption, wondering if this is a means of reducing their benefits, or they may avoid confirming any high-risk areas which can be overcome as they may see this as declaring they are unfit for certain employment.

Given the apparently substantial availability of women's health screening and being in a climate where we are seeking equality for all, the whole area of men's health should be carefully evaluated. The problem lies with the question of who should evaluate the services currently avail-able and how objective would they be? If an audit were carried out to establish what provision is being made nationally, what services are offered and which men are being targeted, the results may depend largely upon who commissioned it.

It is men and men alone who should seek out better health care; they should not need to be cajoled and press-ganged into taking responsibility for their health. Even with women's health screening which was initiated by women for women, there are still women who will not attend for cervical screening or mammography either due to fear or a feeling of 'It will never happen to me'. If this lack of take-up still exists with women then it is only to be expected that men's take-up will be similarly affected. Every opportunity should be taken for advertising well man clinics; they could be advertised in pubs, gyms or garages, anywhere that men can be found. Education relies on the assumption that it is possible to alter the way in which people perceive things by giving them an understanding of ideas and language to rationalize those ideas (Kelly 1992). To hound them and force them into taking up screening and health care is counterproductive and could lead to a more resolute attitude of 'I'll smoke or drink what I like, whenever I like'. It must be done with the consent and full cooperation of each individual and if they have been given the facts and still choose to lead an unhealthy life, that should not be seen as a failure for the providers of health care, who have given thought to targeting, content, venue and timing of clinics to best accommodate men's needs.

REFERENCES

Baker P 1996–7 Men only: is there a role for the well man clinic? Healthlines Dec – Jan: 17–19
Brown I, Lunt F 1992 Evaluating a 'well man' clinic. Health Visitor 1: 12–14
Buetow S A 1996 Testicular cancer: to screen or not to screen? Journal of Medical Screening 3: 3–6
Calman K 1992 Chief Medical Officer's annual report, HMSO
Coulter A, Schofield T 1991 Prevention in general practice: the views of doctors in the Oxford region. British Journal of General Practice 41: 140–143
Deans W 1988 Well man clinics. Nursing 3(26): 975–977
DoH 1992 The health of the nation. HMSO, London
DoH 1995 A whole new ball game. How to check for testicular cancer. Imperial Cancer Research Fund and Department of Health, London
HEA 1994 That's the limit. Health Education Authority, London
Kelly M P 1992 Health promotion in primary care: taking account of the patient's point of view. Journal of Advanced Nursing 17: 1291–1296
Matthews S J 1988 Men and stress. Nursing 3(26): 972–974
Sabo D, Gordon D F (eds) 1995 Men's health and illness. Gender power and the body. Research on men and masculinities. Sage Publications, London
Sadler C 1985 DIY male maintenance. Nursing Mirror (160) 1
UKCC 1997 PREP and you. United Kingdom Central Council for Nursing, Midwifery and Health Visiting, London
Wilson A, McDonald P, Hayes L, Cooney J 1992 Health promotion in the general practice consultation: a minute makes a difference. British Medical Journal 304: 227–230
Wrench J G, Irvine R 1984 Coronary heart disease: account of a preventive clinic in general practice. Journal of the Royal College of General Practitioners September: 477–481

2

Genetic Man

Paul Shilton

INTRODUCTION

Since the dawn of the early primates (approximately 55 million years ago), the development of both the modern-day human male and his female counterpart (i.e. *Homo sapiens*) (Conroy 1990) required a progressive evolutionary divergence from a 'common hominoid ancestor' of *Homo sapiens* and the latter-day species of great apes, i.e. chimpanzees (*Pan troglodytes*), gorillas (*Gorilla gorilla*) and orangutans (*Pongo pygmaeus*). Of interest here, however, is the exclusion of the additional remaining representatives of living hominids, the lesser apes, i.e. gibbons (*Hylobates* spp.) and the siamang (*Symphalangus sydatylus*), as their particular lineage had separated before the subsequent emergence of the 'common hominoid ancestor' to both *Homo sapiens* and the great apes (Relethford 1993).

In view of this, the degree of genetic relatedness between man and each individual member of the great apes can be assessed by comparative analysis of the structural appearance and genetic organization of chromosomes from chimpanzee, gorilla, orangutan and man (Yunis & Prakash 1982). Indeed, the typical constitution of human chromosomes is 46 (the diploid number, consisting of 22 identical or homologous chromosomal pairs with one pair of sex chromosomes) whilst the number associated with the great apes is 48 (the difference from man being an additional associated chromosomal pair) (Fig. 2.1). These are located within the nucleus of all diploid somatic cells (as opposed to the germ cells where the haploid gametes, i.e. male sperm and female eggs, only contain one member of each pair of chromosomes), each chromosome being composed of a highly condensed strand of DNA, deoxyribonucleic acid (the double stranded helical molecule of heredity) which is tightly complexed and subsequently coiled around protective and structurally

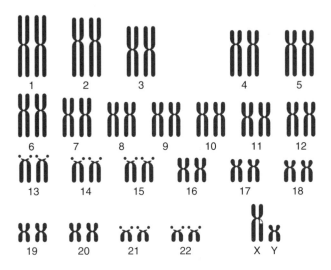

Figure 2.1a Karyotype of human male (note the non-homologous X and Y chromosomes).

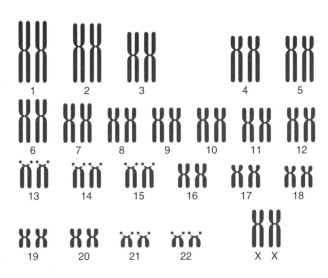

Figure 2.1b Karyotype of human female (note the homologous pair of X chromosomes).

important histone proteins. Further coiling leads to the formation of extraordinarily compact chromosomal chromatin fibres (Fig. 2.2). This brief introduction to chromosomes will be discussed in more detail.

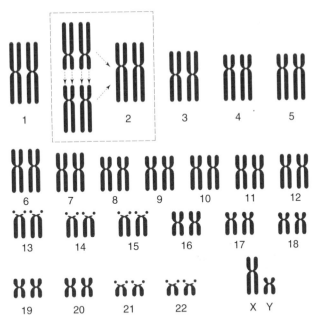

Figure 2.1c Karyotype of a male ape (note the two pairs of homologous acrocentric chromosomes which are believed to have fused together to form human chromosome number 2).

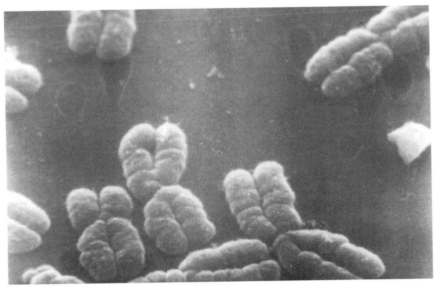

Figure 2.2 Electron micrograph of human chromosomes showing the centromeres and well-defined chromatids. (Courtesy of Dr Christine Harrison. Reproduced from Cytogenetics and Cell Genetics 1983, 35: 21–27 with permission of the publisher, S Karger A G, Basel.)

CHROMOSOMAL SIMILARITY BETWEEN APES AND MAN

Comparison of the chromosomes from man and other primates appears to demonstrate a certain level of relatedness between specific chromosomes from man and each individual member of the great apes, whereby man and chimpanzee have 13 identical pairs of homologous chromosomes, man and gorilla possess nine, whereas man and orangutan share eight. It would be expected that chromosomal similarity is apparent between the great apes themselves and this is indeed the case, e.g. chimpanzees and gorillas share an exclusive combination of 11 chromosomal pairs (Yunis & Prakash 1982). Even so, the apparent differences between the chromosomes of these four species appear to be relatively simple structural changes, the position of certain genes being merely altered within the chromosome. This excludes the possibility of differing chromosomal characteristics on the basis of insertion or deletion of unique gene sequences (Weaver & Hedrick 1991) (the relative severity of these changes thereby reflecting the extent of evolutionary divergence).

By considering these findings with additional comparisons of anatomy (e.g. shared characteristics of the upper body and shoulder; Relethford 1993), biochemistry (e.g. comparing both the structure and the specific amino acid sequences of certain proteins; King & Wilson 1975) and genetics (e.g. DNA-hybridization techniques whereby DNA from two species are exposed to high temperatures in order to separate the two strands of the double helix; the degree of similarity being determined by the extent to which the single strands of the two species reassociate together, the more closely related two species are, the greater the extent of this reassociation; Relethford 1993), it is now possible to speculate upon the common ancestry between man and the great apes and thereby enables a tentative evolutionary pathway to be determined that eventually culminates in the emergence of modern man.

The progressive evolution of ape-like primates is considered to have reached its most significant point during the early period of the Miocene epoch (approximately 16–18 million years ago) when a common ancestor to man and the great apes is believed to have emerged within the varied tropical environments of a fledgling African continent, i.e. open grasslands, savannahs, bushlands and woodlands; the title *Afropithecus* being ascribed to this particular community of early hominoids (based upon geographical distribution and fossil evidence). The separate continents recognized today as Europe and Asia were then joined together, forming a combined area of land known as Eurasia, which subsequently came into contact with the land mass of Africa through continental drift. As a consequence of natural migration, species within the genus *Afropithecus* began to populate southerly regions of both Europe and Asia and subsequently became isolated from those species remaining in Africa. One of these Eurasian species of *Afropithecus* appears to have evolved into a genus known as *Sivapithecus* (approximately 7–14 million years ago) whilst the African members of the genus apparently evolved into a genus called *Kenyapithecus* (14–17 million years ago).

The degree of chromosomal similarity between man and the African apes is apparently greater than that between man and the Asian ape, the orangutan, the suggestion being that *Sivapithecus* was an exclusive precursor to the evolution of the orangutan, whilst *Kenyapithecus* appears to be *the* 'common hominoid ancestor' to man, chimpanzees and gorillas (Yunis & Prakash 1982, Foley 1987, Relethford 1993).

Kenyapithecus was the common ancestor from which the gorilla emerged first. Following the divergence of the gorilla, a final ancestral 'hybrid' remained, this being the subsequent precursor to man and the chimpanzee. However, the eventual appearance of a primitive hominid from which man's evolutionary lineage commenced required a dramatic chromosomal alteration whereby the human diploid complement of 46 chromosomes was achieved following the fusion of one of the 48 chromosome pairs associated with the common ancestor of man and chimpanzee (as well as the modern-day great apes) to form human chromosome 2 (see Fig. 2.1c) (Yunis & Prakash 1982).

It is possible that during this final divergence of chimpanzee and man the fabled 'missing link' between man and the apes may have roamed exclusive regions of the earth (approximately 4–5 million years ago). However, the first hominids belonged to the genus *Australopithecus* (1–4 million years ago) and are believed to have evolved into modern man through a fairly basic sequence. Commencing with the earliest known hominid *Australopithecus afarensis* (dated 3–4 million years ago), several evolutionary pathways developed whereby one particular line led to the progression from *Homo habilis* (1.5–2.4 million years ago) to *Homo erectus* (0.2–1.6 million years ago) to archaic *Homo sapiens* (32 000–200 000 years ago) and ultimately, the anatomically modern *Homo sapiens* (or *Homo sapiens sapiens*; Foley 1987); its appearance dating from 30 000–100 000 years ago to the present day (Relethford 1993).

GENETIC SELECTION

Having established the basic evolutionary development of *Homo sapiens*, the circumstances behind the emergence of such a predominantly influential species can be fundamentally attributed to the strength of genetic selection over successive generations, whereby the continual process of alteration and subsequent expression of man's genotype (the genetic constitution of an individual) has contributed to:

• the phenotypic characteristics (i.e. the physical, biochemical and physiological aspects of an individual as determined by the interaction of his/her genotype and the environment in which it is expressed) observed within various communities following adaptation to a particular environment. For example, global changes in climate can account for the evolutionary selection of different skin colours whereby dark-pigmented skin is prevalent amongst people inhabiting warm tropical equatorial regions, such as Africa (the dark pigment appearing to afford greater protection against exposure to harmful ultraviolet radiation present with a higher intensity of sunlight) while people with light-pigmented skin occupy more temperate regions (individuals with light skin, e.g. Europeans, are less likely to experience injuries, such as frostbite, as a consequence of cold temperatures) (Relethford 1993);

• the superior increase in mental capacity which has enabled the manufacture and use of advanced tools (as opposed to the simple implements utilized by apes) as well as permitting greater proficiency in the use of language and communication;

• the subsequent cultural progression whereby the development of social interaction and social structures has assisted in the ultimate survival of the species.

The expression of the unique genotype associated with a particular individual is directly responsible for their observable phenotypic characteristics and is exclusively determined by the specific molecular structure of DNA contained within the chromosomes of all nucleated cells (Fig. 2.3). Indeed, the chemical and physical nature of DNA is primarily designed to enable an exact sequence of amino acids to be determined, these being required for the construction of both structurally (e.g. collagen) and functionally (e.g. enzymes, such as pepsin which breaks down proteins in the stomach, and hormones, e.g. insulin which regulates the concentration of glucose in the bloodstream) important proteins.

The two intertwined helical strands of DNA are composed of conjoined nucleotides, each nucleotide comprising both a sugar, i.e. deoxyribose,

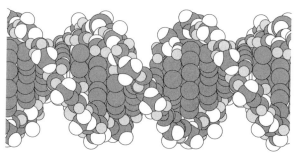

Figure 2.3 The helical double-stranded structure of the gene.

and a phosphate molecule along with one of four distinct nitrogenous bases (the purine bases being known as adenine and guanine and the complementary pyrimidine bases as cytosine and thymine, these being abbreviated respectively as A, G, C and T). The spatial anatomical arrangement of these components creates a deoxyribose-phosphate backbone to each strand, whilst the two chains are held together by specific hydrogen bonding between corresponding pairs of bases (adenine and guanine always being in the opposing chain with thymine and cytosine respectively) which point in towards the centre of the helix (Fig. 2.4).

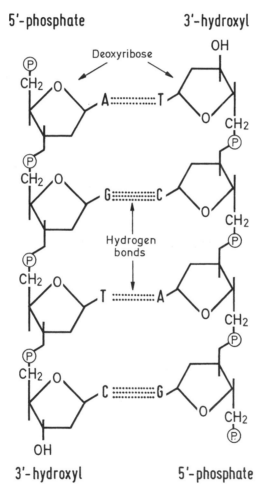

Figure 2.4 Sugar-phosphate backbone and nucleotide pairing of the DNA double helix. P = phosphate; A = adenine; T = thymine; G = guanine; C = cytosine (from Mueller RF, Young ID, 1998, with permission).

These apparently random sequences of nitrogenous bases (occurring along the length of chromosomal DNA) constitute a particular gene and act as a genetic code providing the exact information on the order of amino acids required for the production of a functional gene product. A sequence of three nitrogenous bases (i.e. the triplet codon) is capable of determining one amino acid, e.g. TAC is specific for the amino acid methionine, the overall number of combinations associated with triplet sequences being of sufficient magnitude to ensure that all 20 known amino acids are encoded for, i.e. four bases[3] which permits 64 possible combinations (whereby some amino acids are encoded by a multiple number of triplet base sequences).

The position of a particular amino acid within the primary structure of a polypeptide chain affects both its physical and structural properties, as well as its interaction with surrounding amino acid residues, which can subsequently influence the three-dimensional and functional conformation of the overall protein complex. For example, the amino acid residues of glycine and proline are found predominantly within the internal loop structures of proteins where the structural rigidity of proline imposes a distinctive twist to the polypeptide, while the absence of bulky projections in glycine makes it the only residue which can comfortably occupy the areas of restricted space (Smith 1991).

The progression from genetic information to a functional protein product is the 'central dogma' of molecular biology and involves two important processes, transcription and translation. In the former, the two intertwined strands of DNA temporarily separate so that one of the strands can be utilized as a template (the other becoming inactive) and transcribed into ribonucleic acid, i.e. RNA (in which each nucleotide has a ribose sugar component instead of deoxyribose, while the pyrimidine base thymine is replaced by a thymine derivative known as uracil), whereby free-floating complementary RNA bases are attracted to the single-stranded DNA template. Once this messenger strand of RNA (mRNA) has been formed it separates from the DNA template (thereby allowing the two complementary DNA strands to reanneal) and migrates from the nucleus into the cell's cytoplasmic material, becoming associated with one of the multiple sites of protein synthesis, i.e. the ribosomes.

It is at this point that the information stored within mRNA is translated into a recognizable protein structure, and as such, mRNA becomes a template for another species of RNA known as transfer RNA (tRNA) in which each molecule of tRNA carries both an amino acid and its associated codon, this being complementary to a subsequent codon in the mRNA. As the ribosome traverses along the length of the mRNA strand, successive amino acids are added to a growing polypeptide chain until a stop codon is reached and the completed polypeptide product is released into the cytoplasm (see Fig. 2.5).

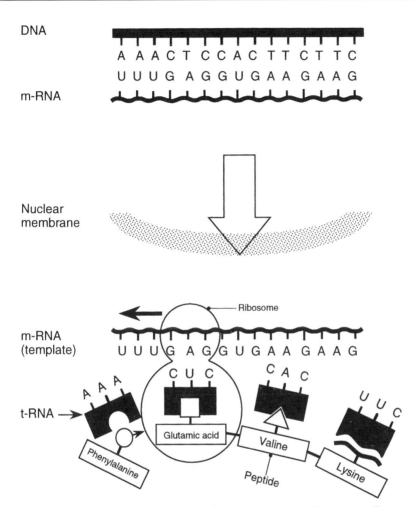

DNA

m-RNA

Nuclear
membrane

m-RNA
(template)

t-RNA →

Figure 2.5   The process by which genetic information is translated into protein (from Mueller RF, Young ID, 1998, with permission).

SEX DETERMINATION MECHANISMS

Having now considered the fundamental mechanism of gene expression and the apparent evolutionary strength of genetic selection, it seems feasible to assume that the development of the male sex within the species of *Homo sapiens* is genetically predetermined and thus genetic expression is directly responsible for the behavioural characteristics of masculinity.

The actual process of sex determination (responsible for the establishment of both males and females within a particular species) appears to involve a variety of distinct methods which can be independently observed in different species and is not therefore regulated by fulfilment of a universal criterion, e.g. environmental factors can influence the sexual orientation of embryonic egg-bound reptiles (i.e. turtles, crocodiles, etc.) whereby exposure to high temperatures produces males in a particular species and females in others (Weaver & Hedrick 1991). However, the sex of most animals is determined at the time of fertilization by chromosomal differences.

As has previously been mentioned, the normal diploid complement of chromosomes within all nucleated somatic cells is 46 and consists of 22 identical or homologous chromosomal pairs with one pair of sex chromosomes. The differentiation between males and females is determined by the particular constitution of these sex chromosomes whereby females possess two homologous X chromosomes (the homogametic sex; 46 XX) whilst males have an unmatched chromosomal pair of one X chromosome and one unique Y chromosome (the heterogametic sex; 46 XY) (see Fig. 2.1a and b).

Having briefly outlined the chromosomal differences between males and females and before explaining the process by which the male sex is determined, it is important at this stage to mention the principles associated with the two principal types of cell division; these being mitosis and meiosis.

Mitosis is the type of somatic cell division that follows fertilization and maintains the diploid complement of chromosomes in successive generations of cell lines whereby genetically identical daughter cells are generated from the genetic duplication and subsequent division of a parental cell. Prior to a cell entering the continuous mitotic process, each strand of chromosomal DNA successfully replicates itself (this arbitrary stage being known as interphase) so that each chromosome consists of a pair of identical sister chromatids joined by a specialized region known as the centromere (this being apparent during prophase). As the chromosomes gradually condense, the nuclear envelope begins to disintegrate and the chromosomes are released into the cytoplasm. Upon liberation, the chromosomes migrate to the equatorial plate of the cell and arrange themselves independently upon a previously formed structure, known as the mitotic spindle, the chromosomes being securely attached by their centromeres to the thin protein fibres that constitute the spindle (metaphase). On contraction of the spindle fibres the centromeres separate, pulling each sister chromatid apart with the two identical daughter chromosomes being drawn to the opposite poles of the cell (anaphase). Once the daughter chromosomes reach the polar ends of the cell, the cytoplasm divides (cytokinesis) whilst the nuclear envelope reforms around each set of uncoiling daughter chromosomes (telophase). As a consequence of this process, two daughter cells are produced, each with an identical genetic constitution (Fig. 2.6).

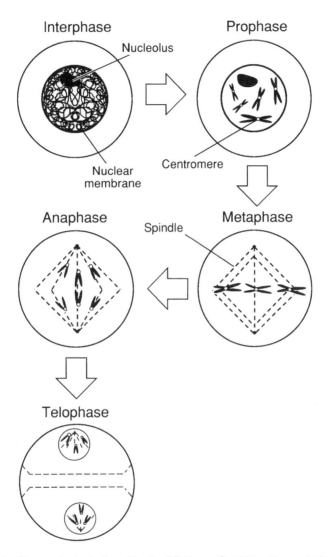

Figure 2.6   Stages of mitosis (from Mueller RF, Young ID, 1998, with permission).

In contrast to mitosis, meiosis occurs exclusively within the germ cells and is characterized by two successive cell divisions (known as meiosis I and II which follow a preceding stage of DNA replication) and is therefore primarily concerned with the formation of the haploid gametes, i.e. male sperm and female egg cells. The diploid number of 46 chromosomes, observed in germline precursor cells, is halved so that the subsequent union of male and female gametes, at fertilization, restores the normal diploid state.

Meiosis also provides an essential and unique opportunity for genetic diversity and this is achieved prior to the first meiotic division, i.e. during meiosis I, when homologous chromosomes (consisting of four chromatids) pair up together and interact to form a bivalent structure (this being unlike the chromosomal independence observed in mitosis). During this stage there is the potential for exchange of genetic material between the chromatids of these non-identical pairs of homologous chromosomes; and as this phenomenon of chiasmata, i.e. the visible areas of chromosomal contact, produces new or recombinant chromosomes. This process also affects the non-homologous X and Y sex chromosomes which, although different, possess homologous or pseudoautosomal regions which enable genetic recombination to occur.

As the reductional meiotic phase of cell division continues each member of the bivalent homologous chromosomal pair separates and migrates to opposing poles of the dividing cell, resulting in the production of two daughter cells each of which having received a haploid set of 23 chromosomes. Shortly after completion of meiosis I, the previously derived daughter cells undergo meiosis II (otherwise known as the equational division) whereby, in a process essentially identical to mitosis, sister chromatids separate at the centromere and migrate into the nuclei of newly dividing daughter cells. As a consequence of this entire meiotic sequence four haploid cells are produced that will subsequently differentiate into four viable spermatozoa (during the testicular process of male spermatogenesis) or a single ovum (via the arduous ovarian process of female ovogenesis, in which the three remaining cells degenerate as non-functional polar bodies) (Fig. 2.7).

Every haploid sperm and egg cell contains 22 autosomes with a single sex chromosome and this is the case for normal female egg cells in which the sex chromosome is always an X. However, the situation in males is slightly more complicated in that, as a consequence of the XY constitution of male sex chromosomes, the meiotic process of spermatogenesis yields sperm of two different types, half carrying an X chromosome and half bearing a Y chromosome. The crucial factor that determines sex is ultimately whether an X or Y-bearing sperm fertilizes the female ovum: a sperm bearing a Y chromosome dictates a male zygote, i.e. fertilized egg, whilst a sperm bearing an X chromosome precipitates the development of a female.

It is interesting at this stage to consider the sex ratio that exists between males and females (highlighting, in particular, those individuals inhabiting industrialized countries) from the time of conception through to the point of old age. Despite the unnerving fact that males are more susceptible to death at almost every stage of life (by virtue of genetic or environmental factors; Waldron 1983), there seems to be an apparent compensatory mechanism in that males have a distinct numerical advantage over females at

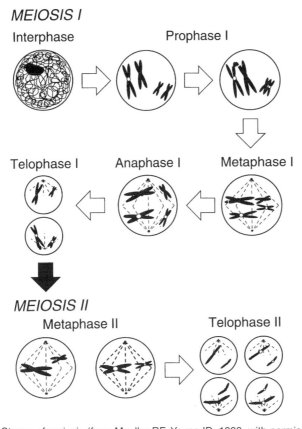

MEIOSIS I

Interphase   Prophase I

Telophase I   Anaphase I   Metaphase I

MEIOSIS II

Metaphase II   Telophase II

Figure 2.7   Stages of meiosis (from Mueller RF, Young ID, 1998, with permission).

the time of both fertilization (primary sex ratio) and birth (secondary sex ratio), this statistical phenomenon being attributed to a variety of plausible causes.

One explanation concerns the efficiency with which Y-bearing sperm appear to reach the awaiting egg before their X-bearing counterparts. Indeed, once the process of coital ejaculation successfully introduces the male sperm into the vagina of the female, the subsequent progress of each genetically rich sperm cell through the mucosa that lines the female genital tract to the fallopian tubes (or oviduct; this being the site where the liberated egg resides) is partly dependent upon the peristaltic muscular contractions within the walls of both the uterus and the fallopian tubes, as well as the rhythmical propulsive undulations of the sperm's own tail. However, the critical advantage associated with Y-bearing sperm is believed to be that the Y chromosome is smaller than the X chromosome and as such the lighter Y-bearing sperm are more mobile than sperm laden with the heavier X chromosome (Singer 1985).

Alternatively, the chemical environment of the female genital tract, both before and during ovulation, can significantly affect the proportions of both X and Y-bearing populations of sperm. The survival of X-bearing sperm is favoured by the acidic nature (i.e. a pH less than 7) of the genital mucosa at approximately 3 days prior to ovulation, while the survival of Y-bearing sperm is enhanced at the point of ovulation when the conditions of the lower genital tract are more alkaline or basic (i.e. a pH between 7 and 14) (Singer 1985).

Once a spermatozoon in prime condition successfully penetrates and fertilizes the female egg (thereby perpetuating the idea of natural selection, whereby the strongest and fittest sperms are associated with genetic superiority), the subsequent union of paternal and maternal sets of chromosomes allows the zygote to undergo a continuous succession of mitotic cell divisions, so that by the time the zygote completes its week-long journey to the uterus it has been transformed into a hollow sphere of genetically identical cells known as the blastocyst. The blastocyst becomes implanted into the lining of the uterus and the embryo then develops into a recognizable fetus by developmental processes involving growth, co-ordinated cellular movements and ultimately cellular differentiation (Roberts 1986).

As the process of embryonic development approaches its sixth week, the sexual nature of the embryo is determined as genetic intervention induces the undifferentiated gonads to fulfil their ovarian or testicular destiny, this apparently being entirely dependent upon the cellular presence or absence of a Y chromosome. The subsequent development of this primitive gonadal tissue into an ovary or a testis is ultimately determined by the coordinated expression of a particular sequence of genes, designated the testis-determining factor (TDF), which is located on the short arm of the genetically inert Y chromosome. In the absence of this genetic region upon the Y chromosome the undifferentiated gonad follows a predetermined pathway of ovarian development, yet in the presence of a Y chromosome this TDF region acts as a genetic switch initiating a 'cascade of processes' (de la Chapelle 1988) that successfully diverts the progress of ovarian gonadal development into a testicular structure which, under the stimulation of human chorionic gonadotrophin (HCG) from the placenta, secretes the male hormones (or androgens) i.e. testosterone and androsterone, that indirectly cause regression of the primitive uterus and fallopian tubes while defining both the internal and external features of masculine genitalia. The continued secretion of these steroid hormones is vital following parturition for they promote growth, activity and further development of the reproductive organs and initiate the masculinizing effects apparent at the time of puberty, i.e. increased growth of facial and body hair, lower pitch of voice, increased muscular definition, increased libido and production of sperm.

Abnormalities of sex determination

Unfortunately, the issue of sex determination is not as simple as this for, in addition to the normal sexual chromosomal constitution of XX (in phenotypic females) and XY (in phenotypic males), there are a small proportion of rare individuals who present as XX males (genotypically female yet phenotypically male), XY females (genotypically male but phenotypically female) and XX true hermaphrodites (in whom the general physique and genitalia appear to display varying degrees of both male and female characteristics, e.g. individuals may possess both a single ovary and a single testicle or a mixture of ovarian and testicular tissue, i.e. ovotestes).

These abnormalities of sexual development can be attributed to an aberration in the process of paternal meiotic recombination (which provides an opportunity for genetic diversity prior to the first meiotic division). Instead of the normal exchange of genetic material between homologous pseudoautosomal regions of the X and Y chromosomes, genetic recombination may occur outside this 'safe' region with the subsequent transfer or translocation of the testis-determining region from the Y to the paternal X chromosome. As a consequence of this, a phenotypic male with a 46 XX karyotype arises following acquisition of the TDF which has been translocated onto a single X chromosome (this also being a possible explanation for XX true hermaphroditism), whilst phenotypic 46 XY females occur because the Y chromosome is affected by deletions or mutations, thereby resulting in the loss of these vital testis-determining sequences. Indeed, a definitive aetiology to account for XX true hermaphroditism may be due to the transferral of male-determining genes onto the paternal X chromosome.

Alternative theories include the possibility of both genetic mosaicism (in which the tissues of a particular individual are derived from a single zygote and present with at least two genotypically different cell lines, e.g. XX/XY) or chimaerism (whereby the differing genotypic cell populations are derived from one or more zygotes). The latter is a consequence of dispermic or blood chimaerism, the former involving the fusion of two independent zygotes, i.e. following the fertilization of two egg nuclei by two genetically different sperm, while the latter arises via the placental exchange of cells between non-identical or dizygotic twins developing in the uterus (Emery & Mueller 1992).

The influence of specific male-determining gene sequences would appear to provide an adequate explanation for all these limited incidences of abnormal sex reversal but there are exceptions to this rule which refute the original theories associated with human sex determination, e.g. the absence of TDF regions in both XX males and XX true hermaphrodites as well as the presence of TDF-containing Y chromosomes in XY females (de la Chapelle 1988). Several alternative hypotheses have been presented which can account for both these abnormal cases of sexual development as well as providing a viable mechanism for the normal process of sex determination.

The first of these particular theories entertains the idea that specific genes may be borne on both the X and Y chromosomes which could each encode for the different subunits of a single dimeric protein (i.e. proteins composed of two subunits whereby each subunit consists of a single polypeptide chain). In consideration of this, cells containing an XY sex chromosomal constitution would produce a heterodimeric (i.e. consisting of two different subunits) testis-determining protein, while cells possessing an XX constitution would encode for a homodimeric (i.e. consisting of two identical subunits) protein to activate the development of ovarian gonadal tissue (de la Chapelle 1988).

However, an even more intriguing possibility could account for the process of sex determination. This is based upon Lyon's hypothesis of X-linked dosage compensation whereby, after approximately 16 days of embryonic development, one of the two X chromosomes within each female somatic cell is randomly inactivated (i.e. the affected X chromosome being of either paternal or maternal origin) and appears as a dark-staining, tightly coiled mass within the nucleus (known as a Barr body). The subsequent expression of X-linked genes on the remaining X chromosomes of descendent cells allows the female's X chromosomal protein products to be generated at an equivalent concentration to those produced by the solitary X chromosomes present within each male. Interestingly, the absence of any X chromosomal inactivation processes would lead to XX female cells producing twice as much of an X chromosomal gene product as that observed in single X males.

The adaptation of this dosage compensation theory as an effective mechanism for the determination of sex therefore encompasses the possibility that there are an equivalent set of genes present on both the X and Y chromosomes which may encode for an identical, yet interchangeable protein product. The subsequent inactivation of a single somatic female X chromosome (in XX females) would result in the production of a single female-determining dose of protein (i.e. following expression of the remaining active X chromosome), while expression of both the X and Y chromosomes (in XY males) would influence the production of a double male-determining dose (Page et al 1987, de la Chapelle 1988).

In view of this dosage compensation model, it is possible to provide an adequate explanation for the normal mechanism of sex determination as well as attributing errors of X chromosomal inactivation to account for the exceptional abnormalities that can affect the sex chromosomes, notable examples being XX males (in whom the Y chromosome is absent) and XY females. In these cases, Y chromosome-deficient XX males experience a failure in the inactivation of the X chromosomal sex-determining locus (a locus simply being the site of a particular gene on a chromosome), so that the subsequent expression of these two active loci results in the phenotypic appearance of a male following the production of a double male-determining dose of protein (German 1988). Alternatively, phenotypic females of an XY sex chromosome constitution endure the normal process of inactivation to the solitary X chromosome so that the subsequent expression of Y-linked genes results in the production of the single female-determining dose of this highly influential, yet undefined protein.

Finally, the extraordinary cases of XX true hermaphroditism can also be explained by variable levels of inactivation of the crucial X chromosomal locus which could account for the contrasting differentiation pattern of sexual embryonic tissue (German 1988, de la Chapelle 1988). Two parental cells within a particular XX hermaphroditic individual could behave according to the following scenario, where one cell undergoes normal inactivation of a single X chromosome to produce a single female-determining dose of protein, while the second cell may suffer incomplete inactivation of the X chromosomal locus, with the subsequent production of a double male-determining dose. As a consequence of this the descendent cells of the developing embryo would differentiate into tissue of both a feminine and masculine nature.

Having concluded this discussion on the factors which may influence the mechanisms of sex determination, it is appropriate to continue with a review of additional sex chromosomal abnormalities (further to those already mentioned) as well as concentrating on the genetic disorders which are considered to exclusively affect the male gender, e.g. colour blindness or haemophilias A and B, etc.

GENETIC DISEASES AND ABNORMALITIES

As has been indicated previously, genetic disease can arise via chromosomal abnormalities which may affect a particular autosome or the sex chromosomes. However, genetic disorders can also occur as a consequence of defects within a single gene, e.g. haemophilia A, or inherited through a multifactorial origin (whereby factors of both a genetic and environmental nature may work in conjunction, e.g. coronary or ischaemic heart disease).

The aetiology of chromosomal abnormalities can be attributed to either a numerical or structural aberration. The former involves the loss or gain of one or two chromosomes (aneuploidy) or even the acquisition of many haploid chromosomal sets (referred to as polyploidy, although both triploidic, i.e. possessing a chromosomal constitution of 69 XXY or 69 XYY, and tetraploidic, i.e. 92 XXXX or 92 XXYY, individuals generally undergo spontaneous abortion during early pregnancy). Abnormalities most commonly encountered with the latter include chromosomal deletions (in which a genetically active segment of a chromosome is lost) and translocations. The reciprocal type of translocation encompasses the exchange of genetic material between homologous or non-homologous autosomes or sex chromosomes, e.g. the previously mentioned transfer of the TDF from the Y to the paternal X chromosome while the Robertsonian type, although not entirely relevant to the sex chromosomes, involves a structural rearrangement between the single members of two different acrocentric chromosomal pairs with the subsequent loss and fusion of small satellite genetic fragments which results in the formation of a fully active chromosomal hybrid (Emery & Mueller 1992) (Fig. 2.8). As a matter of interest, there are an additional series of structural abnormalities which incorporate inversions (in which the position of a particular chromosomal segment is reversed or inverted) duplications (in which a chromosomal segment is represented twice or duplicated), rings (characterized by the deletion of the ends of each chromosome arm with the subsequent fusion of these broken arms, leading to the formation of a ring) and isochromosomes (in which the duplication of a single chromosomal arm, e.g. the long arm, results in the formation of two genetically identical long arms and is followed by the deletion of the opposing arm, e.g. the short arm).

Of the chromosomal abnormalities which can specifically affect the male gender, the most significant include aneuploidic numerical aberrations; for example, trisomy involves the addition of an extra chromosome and is

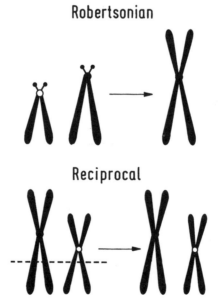

Figure 2.8 Types of translocation (from Mueller RF, Young ID, 1998, with permission).

therefore responsible for the development of a disorder known as Klinefelter's syndrome. Affected individuals usually possess a sex chromosome constitution of 47 XXY and are generally diagnosed during adulthood (i.e. following puberty) upon investigation of infertility since this condition is the single most common cause of hypogonadism and infertility in men (Connor & Ferguson-Smith 1987). Adolescent males present as phenotypically normal but at the onset of puberty, the signs of hypogonadism become more apparent. Affected individuals appear tall and thin (with elongation of the limbs) and the testes remain small (failing to produce the required levels of the masculinizing sex hormones. This subsequently leads to poorly developed secondary sexual characteristics, defective production of spermatozoa (resulting in sterility) and gynaecomastia (excessive growth of the male breast); these symptoms being accompanied by a reduced level of intelligence or mental retardation.

As an alternative to this, a number of clinically asymptomatic individuals have been documented who present with a sex chromosome constitution of 47 XYY (whereby, as in the case of Klinefelter's syndrome, penetration occurs with an incidence of 1 per 1000 male births). This particular karyotype is extraordinary in its association with the development of 'deviant antisocial or delinquent behaviour' (Hook 1973) which correlates with an increased frequency of institutionalization or internment of these individuals (as compared with the incidence in the general XY male population) within various mental or penal establishments (Hook 1973). These individuals are exceptionally tall (tending to reach heights of 6 feet, i.e. 183 cm, and over) and the tendency towards antisocial and delinquent behaviour is considered to be predetermined and independent of environmental factors (such as the rearing of XYY adolescents within deprived socioeconomic backgrounds). Following comparative psychological assessment, the response of delinquency has been attributed to an inability to control aggression (in frustrating and provocative situations), emotional immaturity, impulsive behaviour and a reduced intelligence (Hamerton 1976).

Both of these conditions are consequences of defective segregation of homologous chromosomal pairs during one of the two meiotic cell divisions, this mechanism being referred to as non-disjunction (Fig. 2.9).

As has been mentioned previously, the meiotic segregation of homologous chromosomal pairs results in a haploid set of chromosomes being allocated to each gamete. However, on occasion two of these homologous chromosomes can fail to disjoin, i.e. separate, and may migrate together into the same gamete. This particular error of chromosomal segregation can be effectively illustrated by considering the aetiology of XYY males, in that non-disjunction occurs during meiosis II and results in the formation of gametes that are either lacking any sex chromosomes or have an XX or YY sex chromosome constitution, these chromosomes being exclusively derived from one parent, i.e. of a maternal or paternal origin.

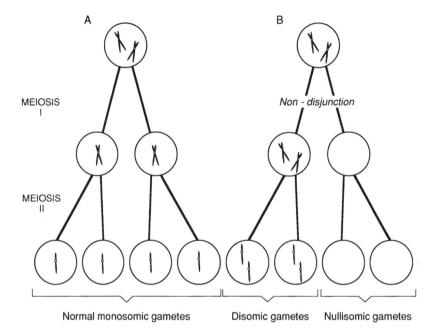

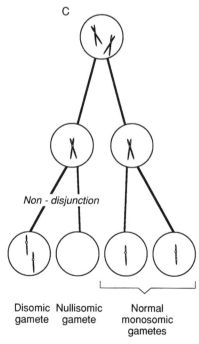

Figure 2.9 Segregation at meiosis of a single pair of chromosomes in (A) normal meiosis, (B) non-disjunction in meiosis I and (C) non-disjunction in meiosis II (from Mueller RF, Young ID, 1998, with permission).

Alternatively, non-disjunction during meiosis I leads to the formation of gametes that, again, lack any sex chromosomes or contain a representative of both the maternal and paternal sex chromosomes, the constitution of these gametes being either XX or XY. Consequently, the subsequent union of an abnormal YY-carrying sperm with a normal X-bearing ovum yields a zygote which possesses an XYY trisomy of sex chromosomes.

Single gene defects

Genetic disorders affecting the male gender also encompass single gene defects whereby a spontaneous or inherited mutation occurs and may subsequently lead to a change in the sequence of the constituent bases of a particular gene (one specific example being point mutations which involve the alteration, insertion or deletion of one or more nitrogenous bases). The subsequent gene product experiences a slight alteration in the sequence of amino acids and this can effectively transform both its structural and functional properties.

The fundamental union of a haploid sperm and egg successfully achieves the desired diploid chromosomal state of the zygote and introduces the 23 paternal chromosomes to their maternal counterparts. However, both the maternal and paternal members of each homologous chromosomal pair contain a strict sequence of equivalent genes. Each individual gene occupies a specific locus upon the chromosomal pair and these alternative forms of genetic information (occurring at a particular locus) are referred to as alleles.

A single gene disorder can therefore be determined by mutation within a specific allele at a single locus on one or both homologous members of an autosomal or sex chromosomal pair (disorders associated with the latter being known as sex-linked, i.e. X-linked or Y-linked). Individuals possessing identical members of a gene pair are termed homozygous (or homozygotes) for that particular locus, heterozygous (or heterozygotes) when the gene pair is different, (i.e. consisting of both a mutant and a normal or wild-type gene, or hemizygous hemizygotes) for individuals who only contain one representative of a homologous chromosomal pair and therefore only possess a single mutant or normal allele. As a consequence of males possessing a single X chromosome a mutant X-linked allele will always be expressed (the male being hemizygous for that allele) for, unlike heterozygous XX females who possess a normal allele, the absence of a normal allele in males fails to counteract the deleterious effect of the mutant allele. These gene-determining characteristics are referred to as dominant, when the trait is typically expressed in the heterozygote, or recessive, when the trait is only expressed in the homozygote, this being apparent as a consequence of the absent masking effect usually provided by a dominant wild-type gene.

There exist five basic patterns of single gene inheritance, of which two in particular, i.e. Y-linked and X-linked recessive, are of most importance to the male gender:

Autosomal dominant

Clinical symptoms are manifest in heterozygous individuals of either sex who generally have one affected parent. There is a 50% chance that the offspring of an affected parent will inherit the trait, e.g. achondroplasia (a skeletal disorder characterized by short-limbed dwarfism and large head) or Huntington's disease (a progressive cerebral degenerative disorder of adult onset characterized by dementia and choreic or involuntary, uncontrollable body movements). Homozygotes for common autosomal traits have been observed in whom the presenting symptoms are of greater severity; however, in the case of rare and more harmful dominant alleles it is assumed that the homozygote state is lethal (Fig. 2.10).

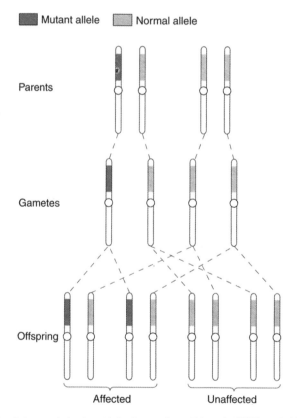

Figure 2.10a Autosomal dominant inheritance (from Edwards CRW et al, 1995, with permission).

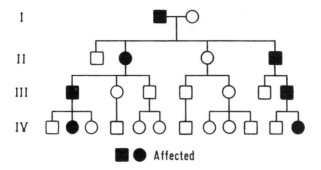

■ ● Affected

Figure 2.10b Family tree of an autosomal dominant trait. □ = male, ○ = female. (From Mueller RF, Young ID, 1998, with permission.)

Autosomal recessive

The clinical symptoms are only apparent in homozygous individuals of either sex (i.e. individuals possessing two mutant alleles, one being situated on each of the two homologous autosomal chromosomes). Both the parents of an affected individual typically present as asymptomatic heterozygous carriers of the mutant allele and each successive mating is associated with a 25% risk of producing an affected homozygote, a 50% chance of conceiving an unaffected heterozygote and a 25% chance that a normal homozygote will be born, i.e. possessing two normal wild-type alleles. However, on occasion, affected progeny can also arise following the rare mating of a heterozygous carrier and an affected homozygote which increases the chances of producing an affected child to 50%, as well as producing a 50% chance of an unaffected heterozygous child (Fig. 2.11).

Autosomal recessive conditions include cystic fibrosis in which the defective transport of sodium and chloride ions, both into and out of epithelial cells, compromises the production of mucus, its high viscosity contributing to chronic pulmonary disease, respiratory infection and pancreatic dysfunction. Sickle cell anaemia (which is believed to confer a selective advantage against the infection of erythrocytes by the malarial parasite *Plasmodium falciparum*), occurs predominantly within Mediterranean, Middle Eastern and Negroid races. The disorder is characterized by the defective production of haemoglobin, i.e. HbA, to yield an alternative structural variant, i.e. HbS, which, under conditions of low oxygen tension, forms insoluble polymers of crystallized haemoglobin, deforming the erythrocyte into the distinctive elongated sickle-shaped cell or drepanocyte (Fig. 2.12). The reduced survival of these red blood cells leads to a chronic haemolytic anaemia, whilst the clumping together of 'sickled' erythrocytes during 'crisis' occludes different regions of the microcirculation, resulting in infarction and necrosis of vital organs and surrounding tissues.

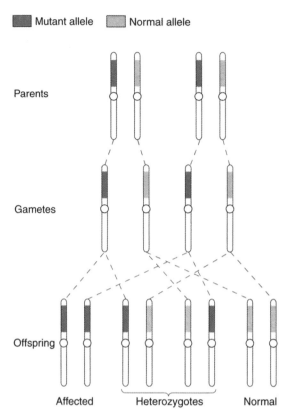

Figure 2.11a   Autosomal recessive inheritance (from Edwards CRW et al, 1995, with permission).

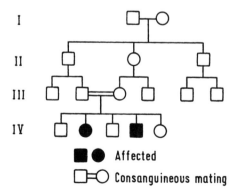

Figure 2.11b   Family tree of an autosomal recessive trait. □ = male, ○ = female. (From Mueller RF, Young ID, 1998, with permission.)

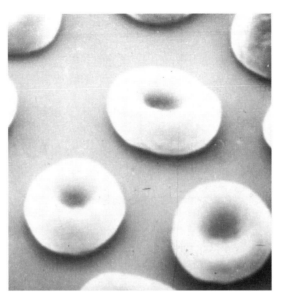

Figure 2.12a Scanning electron micrograph of normal red cells (from Underwood JCE, 1996, with permission).

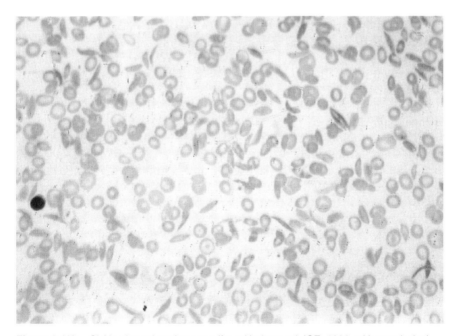

Figure 2.12b Sickle-shaped erythrocytes (from Underwood JCE, 1996, with permission).

Y-linked or holandric inheritance

This pattern of inheritance is associated with genes located upon the Y chromosome and as such, Y-linked traits are only manifest in males, with transmission occurring exclusively between an affected male and all his sons, his daughters remaining unaffected. One of the few examples of Y-linked inheritance is that of maleness, whereby expression of the Y chromosomal TDF initiates the differentiation of the embryonic gonad into a testis. The presence and subsequent expression of this testicular-determining gene accounts for a unique surface antigen, the histocompatibility-Y or H-Y antigen (an antigen being a molecule with specific immunogenic regions that can both stimulate the production of and combine with a specific antibody), detectable upon the somatic and germinal cells of all males. The presence of this H-Y antigen upon somatic cell surfaces provides a reliable indication of maleness and can be utilized when ascertaining the sex of infants whose sex appears ambiguous at birth (Singer 1985). A further, putative example of a Y-linked trait has been observed, known as hairy ear rims. Affected males (commonly originating from populations within the Indian subcontinent) present with long, stiff tufts of hair sprouting from the pinna or rim of the ear.

X-linked dominant

The clinical symptoms for this rare inheritance pattern are typically observed in heterozygous females (in whom the dominant allele is present on one of their two X chromosomes) and hemizygous males (in whom the mutant allele is carried and expressed on the single X chromosome). There is a 50% chance that the offspring of an affected female will inherit the trait. However, as an affected male is only able to transmit this X-linked allele to his daughters (the absence of male-to-male transmission being due to the prospective sons only receiving their father's Y chromosome), there is observed an excess of females e.g., vitamin D-resistant rickets in which, as opposed to the normal aetiology of vitamin D deficiency, the skeletal deformities and weaknesses associated with rickets occur despite an adequate intake of vitamin D and are subsequently found to be refractory (i.e. able to withstand treatment) to therapeutic doses of vitamin D.

X-linked recessive

The phenotypic expression of clinical symptoms typically occurs in hemizygous males (the mutant allele being carried upon the single X chromosome) and, rarely, homozygous females (the recessive alleles being present upon both X chromosomes) (Fig. 2.13). An affected hemizygous

■ Mutant allele   □ Normal allele

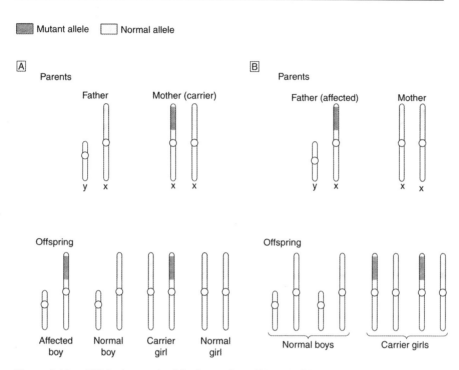

Figure 2.13a   X-linked recessive inheritance (from Edwards CRW, 1995, with permission).

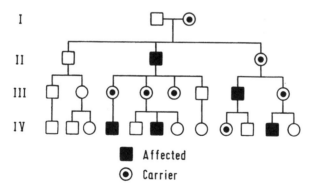

■ Affected
◉ Carrier

Figure 2.13b   Family tree of an X-linked recessive trait in which affected males reproduce (from Mueller RF, Young ID, 1998, with permission).

male arises as a consequence of the mating between an asymptomatic heterozygous female and a normal male, each successive mating being associated with a 25% risk of conceiving a symptomatic hemizygous male, a 25% chance of an unaffected heterozygous female carrier and a 25% chance of producing either a normal male or a normal female. When an affected male reproduces with a normal female the subsequent offspring consist of heterozygous daughters (i.e. carriers of the trait) and unaffected sons. However, in the rare event of the partner being a female carrier (this scenario being possible by virtue of consanguineous relationships, whereby matings occur between related individuals, i.e. first cousins) the subsequent offspring would consist of a potentially extraordinary variety in which there exists a 25% risk of an affected homozygous female, a 25% risk of an affected male, a 25% chance of a heterozygous female carrier and a 25% chance of a normal male.

Examples of X-linked recessive traits include achromatopsia (otherwise known as colour blindness), haemophilias A and B, Becker and Duchenne types of muscular dystrophy, Lesch–Nyhan syndrome, fragile X syndrome and testicular feminization syndrome. These traits are discussed below.

In terms of frequency, *achromatopsia* is one of the most common X-linked recessive traits, with the red-green type of colour blindness being associated with an incidence of approximately 8% of all male births (Emery & Mueller 1992). The normal process of colour perception is dependent upon the differential stimulation of three functionally distinct types of cone, i.e. sensory cells located within the retina of the eye. Each specific cone is more sensitive to absorption of the particular wavelengths of light which corresponds to the blue, green or red region of the visible spectrum. This enables the wavelength of a particular colour to be perceived by the variable stimulation of one, two or all three cone types, e.g. monochromatic blue light is recognized by the exclusive stimulation of the blue cones, whilst the sensation of yellow occurs via the equal stimulation of both the red and green cones (the blue cones remaining inert). Red-green colour blindness occurs because affected individuals lack either red cones (these individuals being referred to as protanopes) or green cones (these being known as deuteranopes). Protanopic individuals perceive a shortened visible spectrum (due to the lack of red cones), whilst deuteranopes possess a fairly normal spectrum, for the absent green cones absorb wavelengths in the middle of the spectrum which can therefore also be absorbed by red or blue cones (Guyton 1981).

The *haemophilias* of type A and B are both congenital disorders which affect the efficient coagulation of blood. Episodes of prolonged bleeding are usually apparent following external trauma or may cause severe internal haemorrhaging, i.e. bleeding within soft tissue. The normal haemostatic response to vascular damage is dependent upon the interaction between the blood vessel or endothelial wall, circulating platelets (or thrombocytes) and blood coagulation factors. The initial adherence of aggregating platelets to the exposed collagen fibres of the endothelial trauma site initiates a complex sequential cascade of enzymic coagulation factor activation, this interactive protein cycle culminating in the formation of a fibrin clot. This insoluble polymer of fibrin strands subsequently strengthens the unstable platelet 'plug' to form a stable fibrin meshwork capable of arresting further loss of blood at the site of injury. Haemophiliacs suffer from a deficiency in the production of a single coagulation factor normally involved in the intermediate steps of the coagulation cascade; the ineffective formation of a fibrin clot accounts for the spontaneous episodes of prolonged bleeding crisis.

Haemophilia A (otherwise known as classic haemophilia) affects approximately 1 in every 10 000 males and is attributed to a deficiency in the synthesis of coagulation factor VIII. The presentation of clinical features is such that affected individuals can be divided according to their respective clinical severity into mild, moderate and severe cases (Antonarakis & Kazazian 1988). Individuals suffering from severe haemophilia experience recurring episodes of spontaneous haemorrhaging into large joints (such as the knees, elbows, ankles and hips, i.e. haemarthroses), whilst muscle tissue is vulnerable to the development of haematomas (i.e. swellings containing blood). The long-term sequelae of haemophilia may involve atrophy (tissue wastage) and necrosis of muscle tissue, swelling and distension within the large joints (synovial hypertrophy), destruction of cartilage and, ultimately, crippling as a consequence of secondary osteoarthritis.

Haemophilia B (otherwise known as Christmas disease) is less common than classic haemophilia, affecting approximately 1 in every 50 000 males (Antonarakis & Kazazian 1988) and is associated with an abnormality of coagulation factor IX. The presentation of symptoms is clinically indistinguishable from those observed in haemophilia A.

The *muscular dystrophies* are a class of hereditary disorders characterized by the progressive weakness, degeneration and atrophy of muscular tissue. In normal individuals a protein known as dystrophin is closely bound with muscle membranes in order to maintain the integrity of the muscle fibre. In affected individuals, the absence of dystrophin leads to the subsequent degeneration of the muscle fibre. However, there are only two forms of muscular dystrophy which are actually associated with an X-linked recessive mode of inheritance and these are the Duchenne and Becker types.

Duchenne muscular dystrophy is the most common type of muscular dystrophy and is associated with an incidence of approximately 1 in 3000 male births. The gradual onset of clinical symptoms usually arises insidiously during early childhood (at approximately 5 years of age) with mild mental retardation, symmetrical muscular atrophy and diminished strength within the thighs and pelvic girdle, as well as enlarged calf muscles (calf pseudohypertrophy). As a consequence, the affected child develops a distinctive waddling action of walking and experiences difficulty in standing up, rising from a sitting position and climbing stairs. As the symptoms of muscle weakness intensify, affected children may be wheelchair bound by the age of 10. Ultimately, they may be confined to bed and they usually die in adolescence (prior to reaching the age of 20).

Becker muscular dystrophy affects approximately 1 in every 20 000 males (Connor & Ferguson-Smith 1987). Following the onset of progressive muscular weakness in late childhood, the presenting clinical features are less severe and so, despite the possibility of wheelchair confinement 25 years after onset, affected individuals generally experience a normal lifespan.

The *Lesch-Nyhan syndrome* affects approximately 1 in every 10 000 males and is caused by the complete deficiency in the synthesis of a single enzyme, hypoxanthine-guanine phosphoribosyl transferase (HPRT), which is required to catalyse the metabolism and subsequent reutilization of preformed purine bases (Stout & Caskey 1988). The clinical symptoms typically associated with abnormal purine metabolism are normally apparent during infancy and may encompass progressive spasticity, postural tremoring and choreoathetosis (an abnormal combination of involuntary, jerky and writhing movements of the hands and feet), a variable degree of mental retardation as well as a characteristically bizarre compulsion towards self-mutilation (biting lips, fingers and the inside of the mouth). The lack of effective therapy against these severe neurological abnormalities results in the eventual death of most sufferers (as a consequence of infection or renal failure) during the second or third decades (Stout & Caskey 1988).

The *fragile X syndrome* is considered to be one of the most common causes of moderate to severe mental retardation and is associated with an estimated incidence of 1 in every 1500 males. As a consequence of a clinically significant 'fragile' site on the long arm of the X chromosome (the chromosome being liable to breakage at this point), the presenting features are classically characterized by a moderate to severe mental retardation, a long head, large ears and a prominent lower jaw (prognathism), large testes (which develop after puberty) and a propensity for epilepsy.

As has been discussed previously, the aetiology associated with the abnormal determination of the male sex is normally attributed to a numerical or structural aberration of the sex chromosomes. However, there exists a particular X-linked recessive form of male pseudohermaphroditism (in which, as opposed to true hermaphrodites, individuals only possess gonadal tissue of the opposite sex) whereby affected individuals are genotypically male (i.e. 46 XY) whilst appearing phenotypically as females. This disorder is known as *testicular feminization* or androgen insensitivity syndrome, with an incidence of approximately 1 in every 20 000 male births. The syndrome appears to be caused by a defect in receptor function so that, despite normal testicular secretion of masculinizing androgens (the testes, in these cases, being located within the abdomen or the groin), there are no corresponding androgen receptors upon the hormones' appropriate target cells and this subsequently prevents the cells' differentiation into functionally active masculine cells. This state of end-organ unresponsiveness to androgens accounts for affected individuals developing the normal physical female characteristics of breasts and external genitalia; the vagina is blind and the uterus and fallopian tubes are absent so these individuals are sterile.

SEXUAL ORIENTATION

Reflecting on the ideas discussed so far, it can be demonstrated that the expression of both normal and defective areas of a particular individual's genotype is the primary determinant in the development of masculine gender.

However, when considering sexual orientation, homosexuality is assumed to be either a matter of choice (conditioned by childhood environment and experiences), genetically determined, e.g. a single gene defect, or even a combination of both genetic and environmental factors (multifactorial inheritance).

Genetic influence upon homosexuality has been supported by a variety of studies (Kallman 1952, Bailey & Pillard 1991, Hamer et al 1993) in which the relative rates of kinship homosexuality (where homosexuality is apparent amongst brothers of the same generation) were shown to be greater between monozygotic twins, i.e. identical twin brothers who are both homosexuals, dizygotic or fraternal twins, i.e. non-identical homosexual twins, and sibling or biological non-twins, than those observed in genetically unrelated or adoptive brothers. The estimation subsequently derived from this is that brothers of male homosexuals are approximately 4–5 times as likely as heterosexual controls to be homosexual (Pillard & Weinrich 1986). Furthermore, additional pedigree analysis of the families of homosexual individuals reveals more homosexual relatives on the maternal side than on the paternal side: homosexuality was found to be more common among maternal uncles and sons of maternal aunts, i.e. cousins, than is normally associated with heterosexuals in the general population. The implication is that a theoretical homosexual trait may be exclusively inherited on the X chromosome by female family members and that the genetic determinants of homosexuality could be acquired via an X-linked mode of inheritance (Hamer et al 1993).

Further research has isolated a chromosomal region, known as Xq28, situated at the tip of the long arm of the X chromosome which may contain a gene (or genes) that influences male sexual orientation (Hamer et al 1993).

The anatomical differences observed between males and females, in both the physical dimensions of their body and brain sizes, are well documented (e.g., on average, male brains are slightly larger than females' and, as most women would probably testify, more dense). However, measurable anatomical differences have also been observed between the brains of heterosexual and homosexual males.

The particular region of cerebral importance concerns a certain group of cells, known as INAH3 (derived from 'third interstitial nucleus of the anterior hypothalamus'), located within the medial preoptic region of the hypothalamus (Levay & Hamer 1994). This region in males is approximately three times larger than in females, however, this difference is also observed between heterosexual and homosexual males; the region in heterosexuals is up to three times larger whilst the homosexual region is of comparable size to that of a female and, in some cases, may be absent altogether (Levay 1991).

It can be postulated that the expression of specific genetic sequences, implicated in homosexuality, initiates the production of certain neurohormones which subsequently affect the degree of masculinization and defeminization of the hypothalamus during the early periods of sexual differentiation and prenatal brain development (Bailey & Pillard 1991).

It is interesting to consider how these genetically inferior homosexuality genes could persist within the population gene pool despite the overwhelming action of evolutionary counterselection; this apparent genetic inferiority being due to the infrequent sexual relationships between females and homosexual males. The subsequent reduction in the reproductive rate of homosexual males leads to the conception of fewer children, contrasting with the genetic fitness of their heterosexual counterparts.

One explanation, originally suggested by Hutchinson (1959; cited by Wilson 1975), is that these homosexual genes are superior in the heterozygous state. However, the exclusive expression within males who have a low reproductive rate suggests that evolutionary survival must require inheritance from female family members (thus accounting for the large proportion of homosexual relatives on the maternal side) (Levay & Hamer 1994). Alternatively, homosexual members of primitive societies may have functioned as helpers, acting as hunting companions, providing domestic support or assisting close relatives, and so, if selection helped to secure the welfare and ultimate survival of the community then genes favouring homosexuality could be sustained within the population by kin selection alone (Wilson 1975).

Unfortunately, various authors sympathetic with the 'gay' campaign for equal rights choose to discredit the current research isolating a gene (or genes) for homosexuality. They believe that the discovery of a gene that predisposes individuals to homosexuality could lead to the development of prenatal diagnostic tests which would enable heterosexual couples to decide whether or not they wished to abort a homosexual foetus (Watney 1995), thereby pandering to the will of a hidden political eugenic policy.

The gender differences observed between the physical, psychological and behavioural aspects of both males and females are largely considered to be culturally determined. However, this discussion has supported the possibility of gender differences being apparent as a consequence of genetic expression. This belief in genetic determinism is strengthened by a recent study assessing the cognitive function in females suffering from Turner's syndrome (a sporadic chromosomal disorder in which all or a section of one X chromosome is absent); the findings reflecting the differences in male and female social cognitive skills. The paternally derived X chromosome appears to possess a genetic locus (situated close to the central or centromeric region) which, when expressed in females, is believed to influence the development of refined social functioning and related cognitive abilities (McGuffin & Scourfield 1997), thereby accounting for the phenomenon of female intuition, whilst the inactivity of this genetic region in males increases the likelihood of social ineptitude, unawareness and disruptive behaviour (Skuse et al 1997).

CONCLUSION

It can be concluded from this that the various facets of masculinity are genetically determined. However, the evolutionary process of natural selection maintains successful genes within the population gene pool (at the expense of genes of inferior genetic fitness) and the genetic influence upon behavioural characteristics both initiates and develops the cultural and environmental factors which may subsequently alter an individual's genetic constitution (i.e. following mutations, etc). This can affect the evolutionary progress of the male gender and, ultimately, that of mankind as well.

REFERENCES

Antonarakis S E, Kazazian H H 1988 The molecular basis of hemophilia in man. Trends in Genetics 4(8): 233–237
Bailey J M, Pillard R C 1991 A genetic study of male sexual orientation. Archives of General Psychiatry 48: 1089–1096
Connor J M, Ferguson-Smith M A 1987 Essential medical genetics, 2nd edn. Blackwell Scientific Publications, London
Conroy G C 1990 Primate evolution. W W Norton, New York
de la Chapelle A 1988 The complicated issue of sex determination. American Journal of Human Genetics 43: 1–3
Edwards C R W, Bouchier I A D, Haslett C, Chilvers E R 1995 Davidson's principles and practice of medicine. Churchill Livingstone, Edinburgh
Emery A E H, Mueller R F 1992 Elements of medical genetics, 8th edn. Churchill Livingstone, Edinburgh
Foley R 1987 Another unique species: patterns in human evolutionary ecology. Longman Group, Harlow

German J 1988 Gonadal dimorphism explained as a dosage effect of a locus on the sex chromosomes, the gonad-differentiation locus (GDL). American Journal of Human Genetics 42: 414–421

Guyton A C 1981 Textbook of medical physiology, 6th edn. W B Saunders, London

Hamer D H, Hu S, Magnuson V L, Hu N, Pattatucci A M L 1993 A linkage between DNA markers on the X chromosome and male sexual orientation. Science 261: 321–327

Hamerton J L 1976 Human population cytogenetics: dilemmas and problems. American Journal of Human Genetics 28: 107–122

Hook E B 1973 Behavioural implications of the XYY genotype. Science 179: 139–150

Kallman F J 1952 Twin and sibship study of overt male homosexuality. American Journal of Human Genetics 4: 136–146

King M C, Wilson A C 1975 Evolution at two levels: molecular similarities and biological differences between humans and chimpanzees. Science 188: 107–116

Levay S 1991 A difference in hypothalamic structure between heterosexual and homosexual men. Science 253: 1034–1037

Levay S, Hamer D H 1994 Evidence for a biological influence in male homosexuality. Scientific American 270(5): 20–25

McGuffin P, Scourfield J 1997 A father's imprint on his daughter's thinking. Nature 387: 652–653

Mueller R F, Young I D 1998 Emery's elements of medical genetics. Churchill Livingstone, Edinburgh

Page D C, Mosher R, Simpson E M et al 1987 The sex-determining region of the human Y chromosome encodes a finger protein. Cell 51: 1091–1104

Pillard R C, Weinrich J D 1986 Evidence of familial nature of male homosexuality. Archives of General Psychiatry 43: 808–812

Relethford J H 1993 Fundamentals of biological anthropology. Mayfield, Mountain View

Roberts M B V 1986 Biology: a functional approach, 4th edn. Thomas Nelson, Walton-on-Thames

Singer S 1985 Human genetics: an introduction to the principles of heredity, 2nd edn. W H Freeman, New York

Skuse D H, James R S, Bishop D V M et al 1997 Evidence from Turner's syndrome of an imprinted X-linked locus affecting cognitive function. Nature 387: 705–708

Smith C A 1991 Globular proteins. In: Smith C A, Wood E (eds) Biological molecules. Chapman and Hall, London

Stout T J, Caskey T C 1988 The Lesch–Nyhan syndrome: clinical, molecular and genetic aspects. Trends in Genetics 4(6): 175–178

Underwood J C E 1996 General and systematic pathology. Churchill Livingstone, Edinburgh

Waldron I 1983 Sex differences in human mortality: the role of genetic factors. Social Science and Medicine 17 (6): 321–333

Watney S 1995 Gene wars. In: Berger M, Wallis B, Watson S (eds) Constructing masculinity. Routledge, New York

Weaver R F, Hedrick P W 1991 Basic genetics. Wm C Brown, Dubuque

Wilson E O 1975 Sociobiology: the new synthesis. Harvard University Press, Cambridge, Mass

Yunis J J, Prakash O M 1982 The origin of man: a chromosomal pictorial legacy. Science 215: 1525–1530

3

Men's health and culture

Howard Shilton

Introduction	Male gender culture
Cultural diversity	Male gender and health
Enculturation	Postmodern man
Gender type	Conclusion
Morbidity and mortality	

INTRODUCTION

The way the concept of culture is used varies depending upon the form of discourse in which it is employed. Within public discourse it is used as a somewhat vague notion to do with the development of the mind and manners; the phrase 'a cultured person', for example, tends to be an indication of such factors as intellect, bearing, polite and social interaction and, in particular, knowledge of and an appreciation of the 'arts'. In other words, to be 'cultured' is to be 'civilized'. The greatest civilizations are the most prolific and advanced in the arts and are referred to as 'the great cultural centres of the world – Paris, London, Venice' (Hodin 1972). Indeed, Hodin argues that the 'artist is the most sensitive tentacle of mankind in its encounter with the complexities of life'. Thus, from Hodin's point of view, art is the pivotal centre of culture.

In professional discourse the sociologist's or indeed the social anthropologist's conceptualization of culture, although perhaps lacking in precision, is more clearly defined. Generally speaking, 'Culture refers to the whole way of life of the members of a society' (Giddens 1989). Helman (1994) builds upon E. B. Taylor's 1871 definition: 'That complex whole which includes knowledge, belief, art, morals, law, custom, and any other capabilities and habits acquired by man as a member of society', and R. M. Keesing's 1981 definition that cultures are: 'systems of shared ideas, systems of concepts and rules and meanings that underlie and are expressed in the ways that human beings live'. From these definitions, Helman postulates that culture is both implicit and explicit guidelines that tell members of a particular society how to 'view the world' and how to 'behave in it'. Helman stresses that these guidelines are inherited by the use of symbols, language, art and ritual.

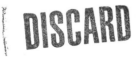

CULTURAL DIVERSITY

Carrithers (1992) points out the importance of recognizing the magnitude of cultural differences given the diversity of human life. Human ways of living are not homogeneous and the resultant cultural diversity may be reflected in factors such as gender role, language, diet, dress, livelihood, domestic organization, religion and cosmological beliefs. Thus, epidemiologically it is possible to consider cultural diversity in relationship to a specific cultural factor such as diet or gender role. Both of these cultural factors may be shown to be implicated in disease or illness causation; for example, in the former case, rickets in South Asian immigrants to Britain, gastric carcinoma in the Japanese, ischaemic heart disease in the British. In the latter case, the traditional male gender role predominant in Western culture may be implicated in stress-related conditions such as primary hypertension.

However, in considering cultural diversity, it is worthy of note that individuals from distinct cultures who have migrated to another country may undergo some degree of acculturation, whereby they adopt some of the cultural aspects of the majority host culture along with the concomitant culturally associated diseases and illnesses. An example of this is that male Japanese migrants to the West who adopt a Western diet and a stress-sensitive lifestyle tend to have an increased incidence of ischaemic heart disease (Marmet & Syme 1976). Helman (1994) emphasizes the point that those migrants who retain a traditional Japanese lifestyle show a lower incidence of ischaemic heart disease.

It is therefore reasonable to conclude that a person's cultural background may have considerable epidemiological significance, the precise nature of which is dependent upon the specific culture or the particular facet of a culture. Adherence to a particular cultural facet, such as the 'keep fit' culture, may contribute to what is perceived to be healthy or, conversely, what is perceived to be unhealthy, such as the 'smoking' culture. Disease and illness may also be viewed as being culturally specific in that they present as unique to a particular cultural group. Examples of these 'culture-bound disorders' include obesity and, paradoxically, anorexia nervosa in the West and cannabis psychosis in Rastafarian West Indians.

ENCULTURATION

Different cultures are separated by boundaries and may be shown to be clearly or somewhat vaguely distinct. Cultural boundaries take the form of territorial boundaries delimiting geographical identity, whereas ideological and behavioural boundaries include such factors as political and social organization and roles within society, kinship systems and gender roles and how the rules, beliefs and mores of a particular culture are transmitted. The process of enculturation, whereby a person learns or is socialized into a culture, is seen by Helman (1994) as the acquisition of a 'cultural lens' in that an individual's perception and understanding of the world are formed, shaped and established and consequently maintain cultural cohesion and continuity.

It follows, then, that the transmission of culture or cultural patterning is a process that is socially determined rather than biologically determined. In other words, a specific cultural lens is not an inborn product of nature. This can be illustrated by considering the universal acquisition of language. The ability to assimilate and utilize a spoken language is a relatively rapid development in a child irrespective of which culture a child is born into. The fact that different cultures have evolved different languages clearly demonstrates that languages are a construction of their respective cultures and as such are socially determined. Furthermore, different forms of language can be demonstrated in single cultures. Bernstein (1971), for example, has shown that in the British culture different language forms can be related to social stratification, in that a 'restricted code' characterized by its grammatically limited, syntactically poor short sentences is predominantly used by the working class and is also accessible to the middle class, whereas the 'elaborated code' characterized by accurate grammatical and syntactical structure and extended sentences is almost exclusively used by the middle class. These observations lend further support to the point that language forms are socially and culturally constructed. This is not to say that biological determinism is not involved, for it can be argued that whilst language forms and usage are culturally constructed, the actual ability to make vocal and verbal utterances in the first instance is a biological phenomenon.

It is accepted that we are born with anatomical structures and a neural organization that enable us to vocalize and verbalize. According to Chomsky (cited by Aitchison 1976), the capacity for language is dependent upon a hypothetical inborn facility referred to as the 'language acquistion device' which provides a child with the biological potential for linguistic skill. Thus the unique human phenomenon of language illustrates a sociocultural-biological dichotomy in that biology determines the capacity for language whilst sociocultural factors determine language form and usage.

Similarly, the absolute need for human nutrition is biologically determined, whereas the form and type of diet taken and the way food is produced, prepared and consumed are socially and culturally determined. Interestingly, Dawkins (1997), in discussing the humble fig, presents the concept of the sociocultural-biological dichotomy by pointing out that the fig can be viewed from a botanical perspective, which concerns its structural detail and its natural history, or from a sociocultural perspective which concerns the fig as metaphor, the fig as symbol and the correct way a fig should be eaten in 'society'. If the sociocultural-biological dichotomy argument is accepted then it follows that the human male can be viewed from the same stance as the fig, so that the biological perspective of the male concerns specific anatophysiological detail, whereas the sociocultural perspective concerns what is perceived to be the correct way for a male to 'view the world' and 'behave in it' in a given culture. In other words, biology determines the male sex or genetic gender, whereas culture determines the male social gender role. In terms of belief and behaviour, therefore, the human male is a sociocultural construction and as such is subject to sociocultural influence on percep-tions, attitudes and responses to health, ill health and health care.

GENDER TYPE

Gender occupies a central position in culture in that gender type, as a pivotal phenomenon, largely directs what gendered individuals believe and how they behave. All cultures, irrespective of geographical location or technological and intellectual advancement, classify people by gender, namely male and female, and the sociocultural division of people into gender type results in the respective 'gender cultures' whereby males and females are encultured and socialized to develop their respective gender identities and conform to gender role expectations. Thus, the biologically gendered male becomes the socioculturally gendered male whereby biological gender type, in most cases, is a sociocultural signal for rather than a cause of the male social gender role.

Within Western culture gender tends to be viewed as a composition of elements which are described by Helman (1994) as the 'components of gender', consisting of genetic, somatic, social and psychological dimen-sions. Genetic gender refers to the genetic composition or genotype of an individual and is represented by X and Y chromosomal presentation, XY being male, XX being female, whereas somatic gender refers to the phys-ical characteristics or the phenotype of an individual and is particularly concerned with the development of the secondary sex characteristics associated with sexual maturity. The genetic and somatic components of gender are clearly anatophysiobiochemical in character and as such are biologically determined. The social gender, however, is socioculturally determined and refers to the way an individual is framed into a gender type in which there is an expectation that they will feel and behave in accordance with a gender culture; thus, there is a general expectation for men to be tough, combative and competitive.

In respect of social gender, Douglas (1973) has postulated that individ-uals consist of two bodies: the social body and the physical body. Douglas argues that the social body constrains how the physical body is perceived and experienced. Therefore combative, competitive and risk-taking behaviour as perceived, experienced and exhibited in the male physical body is socioculturally constructed. Douglas also argues that there is a concordance of expression between the two bodies so that each reinforces the other. The body therefore acts as a symbol and as an expression of meaning, it expresses social pressure and cultural patterning which determines the pattern of male gender behaviour. In this respect Mauss (1973), in his seminal work on behaviour, proposed that there is no such thing as a natural behaviour. All human behaviour, which he referred to as 'techniques of the body', are learnt, providing people with social gender identity and governing such activities as talking and walking, the implication being that all male social gender behaviour concerning and affecting health, ill health and health care is culturally constructed or learnt.

The final gender component, the psychological gender, concerns an individual's self-perception of their genetic identity and introduces Scheper-Hughes & Lock's (1987) concept of the 'mindful body'. These authors point out that emotion is by necessity a component of the mindful body and as such exerts an influence on the way in which engendered self-identity and indeed health and ill health are experienced. It is a pertinent and generally accepted point that the gender components of an individual may present as anomalous and ambiguous; for example, an individual may be genetically and somatically male and may present the embodiment of a male in response to societal expectations, yet in terms of psychological gender may 'mindfully' perceive themselves to be essentially female. Such a situation may lead to difficulties of a medicosocial nature ranging from conflict and discordance in relation to male social gender role expectation to the overt embodiment of female sexuality. In terms of societal expectations of male behaviour as a reflection of 'manhood' within the male gender role, there would seem to be a considerable difference, to use the words of Herzfeld (1985), between 'being a good man' and 'being good at being a man'.

MORBIDITY AND MORTALITY

Demographic research tends generally to show higher levels of morbidity and mortality in men. Interestingly, this demographic phenomenon is graphically illustrated by Grayson (1990) whose analysis of the morbidity rate and mortality rate during the Donner party expedition of 1846–47 reveals a representative microcosm of contemporary society. These findings demonstrate the factors that affected survival for the Donner party, but also reflect current gender-related morbidity and mortality figures, suggesting, as Brannon (1996) points out, that Grayson's analysis gives as much information about current lifestyles and gender roles in relation to men's health as it does about events 100 years ago.

During the summer of 1846, 87 members of the Donner party travelling from Illinois to California utilized an untested route and, due to delays, became stranded in the heavy winter snows of the Sierra Nevada. Forty members of the party had died by the time the survivors were rescued. Most interestingly, in terms of men's health as an aspect of natural selection in action, Grayson's analysis strongly indicates that survivorship was mediated by gender and social factors. As regards gender, the mortality rate in men was significantly higher than in women and furthermore, men tended to succumb sooner and at a higher rate to the vagaries of the harsh conditions. The reference to social factors in Grayson's analysis refers, first, to lifestyle and the male gender role and, second, to social network theory. It is a cogent argument that the male social gender role expectation meant that the adult male members of the party felt obliged to perform tasks associated with short-term physical exertion, thereby increasing their vulnerability to cold and hunger. Also of interest in respect to the male lifestyle, four men died of active or passive violence whereas none of the women's deaths were reported to be as a consequence of violence. The second factor, social network theory, presents the notion that an inverse relationship exists between two variables: mortality and the degree of participation in social networks usually recognized as kin groups. In other words, reduced mortality rates can be demonstrated in those individuals with larger kin groups.

The point to be made from the analysis of the Donner party expedition is that levels of mortality and morbidity in the adult male are directly influenced by the combative and competitive lifestyle and the traditional male social gender role which is essentially a product of sociocultural patterning. Furthermore, mortality is further influenced by kin group size in the sense that kin groups provide an infrastructure of support in times of stress and ill health, a point which is perhaps of some significance in respect to the modern nuclear family. The inference made by Grayson, certainly worthy of reiteration, is that contemporary studies of male mortality and morbidity support the findings of the Donner expedition analysis.

MALE GENDER CULTURE

The social gender role as a cultural construction can be viewed as something of a dramaturgy in the sense that the word 'role' is, according to Brannon (1976), historically derived from the French for 'roll', meaning the roll of paper on which an actor's part was printed. Therefore, from a social perspective both the male and female gender role is performed as culturally scripted, fulfilling the requirements of the part in acting masculine or feminine as appropriate. Thus, to act the expected masculine role is to behave within the dominant cultural paradigm that, ironically, may or may not differ from the 'actual' personality of the theatrical or social actor. Such 'scripted' patterns of behaviour associated predominantly with one gender and not the other, such as repairing a car engine, have led to the formulation of the rigid gender stereotypes that represent a polarity of men's and women's interests. Lewin (1984) refers to this divergence of interest as the 'doctrine of two spheres', generally demonstrating separate spheres of influence as the home and children for women and the outside world and work for men. Thus, it is usual to expect women to be considerably more concerned with personal and family health and health care than men. This highly stereotypical viewpoint forms the basis for the traditional social gender role and, furthermore, as Lewin points out, acts as a social tool for the measurement of masculinity and femininity.

The general traits and characteristics of the traditional male gender role are described by various commentators (Pleck 1976, Helman 1994, Brannon 1996) as being combative and competitive, physically active and strong, coarse and independent. Although these characteristics are predominantly physical in composition, Pleck (1976) presents an essential paradox within the role in that in contemporary society there is an ever-increasing expectation of intellectual and interpersonal competencies, giving rise to the 'modern man' emerging from the traditional paradigm. In the modern male gender role, cognitive abilities and interpersonal skills are positively sanctioned in that they promote achievement in powerful and influential areas of contemporary society, such as medicine, management and academia. Also, there is an expectation that the capacity for emotional intimacy, tenderness and companionship is evident in relationships with women. However, as Pleck argues, the situation is not that men used to have traditional roles and now have modern roles. Rather, the modern role has evolved as an aspect of a dynamic and shifting culture. Yet the physicality of the traditional role persists in the personalities of 'modern man' and is evident in the form of the 'real man' phenomenon whereby men admire and aspire to be like male icons such as Clint Eastwood (Horrocks 1995) and seek compensatory experiences that offer masculine validation such as physical contact sports and risk-taking behaviour.

MALE GENDER AND HEALTH

It is therefore the traits and characteristics of the traditional male gender role with an admixture of cognitive elements and sensitivity that have produced the modern male gender role. Furthermore, it can be said that the modern male gender culture consists of a number of factors that can be considered to be directly or indirectly contributory to men's ill health. In other words, the male gender culture in many aspects is pathogenic rather than protective of health and the majority of the negative aspects can be categorized under the rubric of 'lifestyle choices and occupation'.

In respect to lifestyle, it would appear that the excesses of smoking, alcohol and diet are active variables in ill health causation. Helman (1994) points out that in comparison with women, men are actively encouraged to drink more alcohol and smoke more cigarettes, both activities being a validation of masculinity, 'oiling the social wheels' of male bonding. It is well documented that smoking directly contributes to bronchitis, emphysema, bronchogenic carcinoma and ischaemic or coronary heart disease and that alcohol directly contributes to hypertension and can lead to alcoholism and its associated physical diseases and indirect social consequences.

As regards diet, Brannon (1996) argues that children are generally encouraged to eat a high-protein, high-carbohydrate diet and that this tends to be continued into adult life in men but usually undergoes a fine adjustment in adolescent women. According to Green (1987), it is a general truism that men *do* eat more than women. It is interesting to note that in Green's study, non-participant observation revealed that men ate more because they simply took bigger bites, the reason put forward for this phenomenon being that to eat less and to take small bites is in the male collective psyche considered to be a feminine trait. The inherent problems associated with dietary excess over a prolonged period of time are clear; they include obesity and its concomitant problems of a tendency to heart failure and diabetes mellitus, for example. Also of relevance is the type of diet taken, diets high in animal fats and low in fruit and vegetables being strongly associated with ischaemic heart disease and carcinoma of the colon respectively. A diet high in red meat and the so-called 'junk foods' and low in so-called 'rabbit food' tends to be encouraged by the male gender culture – hence the popularity of the advertising slogan of the 1980s: 'Real men don't eat quiche'.

In the male gender culture there are a number of activities that validate masculinity that may be described as risk-taking behaviour and are almost exclusively considered to be male pursuits. Helman (1994) stresses that, as a consequence of such behaviour, men's health, particularly that of younger men, is often put at risk and indeed is often subject to moderate to severe or fatal injury by dangerous, combative and competitive activities and sports, examples including high-speed and reckless driving, playing rugby and soccer hooliganism. A further cultural factor of considerable significance is that men, by virtue of their occupations, may be exposed to risk situations that potentially may cause injury or ill health. In the former case, it may involve an accident with machinery leading to the loss of a limb, for example, or in the latter case exposure to substances in the working environment such as asbestos leading to asbestosis or coal dust leading to pneumoconiosis. As a further example, high workloads and difficult management situations may lead to stress in the stress-prone individual, contributing to mental ill health or ischaemic heart disease.

Research tends to indicate that the susceptibility of men to ischaemic heart disease is mediated by sociocultural factors. Friedman & Rosenman (1959), in a seminal work on the subject (more recently discussed in Rosenman 1978), introduce what they refer to as the type A behaviour pattern, strongly suggesting that this type of behaviour pattern and personality type has an increased risk of developing ischaemic heart disease in comparison to type B behaviour pattern, the converse of type A. Waldron (1978), in considering the type A behaviour pattern in men, has concluded that whilst susceptibility to ischaemic heart disease may be partly due to biochemistry, sociocultural factors, specifically type A behaviour, also contribute to its aetiology.

The characteristics of the type A behaviour pattern are described by Waldron (1978) as 'hard driving' in nature, and include such factors as ambition, need for professional success, competitiveness, aggressive approach to work and to life in general, work orientation with family and leisure being less important, chronic impatience and an obsession with time. Two points of interest are worthy of note. First, these characteristics clearly show some similitude to the stereotyped male gender role behaviour, an observation, points out Harrison (1978), that was not noted by the researchers who developed the type A and B behaviour construct. Second, type A behaviour in contemporary industrial society is rewarded with professional success and is therefore reinforced and encouraged by the male gender culture. Indeed, men who exhibit type A behaviour frequently become established as successful executives, politicians and senior managers. As a reflection of this successful pathway, Helman (1994) suggests that parents and secondary socializing agencies are likely to promote type A behaviour in boys, thus perpetuating the sociocultural construct.

In many non-industrial societies type A behaviour pattern rarely develops (Waldron 1978), possibly because the work culture within a rural society tends to be mediated by the rise and fall of the sun and the pace of life is regulated accordingly. In industrial society, however, the population has evolved into an 'urban species' in that the work culture is ruled by a culturally constructed time system, in which people are expected to complete high-performance tasks within a 'time urgency' frame. In such a scenario, type A behaviour tends to be rewarded with success, thus reinforcing and perpetuating the construct. It is therefore reasonable to support the viewpoint that type A behaviour pattern is a Western 'culture-bound syndrome', being almost exclusively a construct of the cultural values of contemporary industrial society and an embodiment of the frenetic daily life of an 'urban society'.

A further negative aspect of the male gender culture is the phenomenon of professional health care avoidance. It is a generally held view, that tends to be supported by survey research, that women report symptoms of illness, seek the help of a doctor and utilize hospital services significantly more than men (Mechanic 1978). This is supported by Whitehead (1988) who states that women consistently seek professional help for episodes of acute and chronic illness whereas men do not. This does not necessarily mean, however, that there are higher levels of morbidity among women but that illness among men may simply not be reported.

In terms of the normal iatrogenic sequence (Frankenburg 1980) of illness (the subjective embodiment of ill health; Shilton 1996), followed by the socializing of the illness (i.e. sickness) and finally disease (the basic biomedical entity of ill health; Shilton 1996), the second and final elements are absent and technically therefore do not exist. In other words, individuals avoiding health care may be subjectively aware of their potential or actual ill health and technically therefore will have an illness, yet if they choose not to socialize their illness by not consulting a doctor, then a diagnosis will not be made and consequently a disease will not be revealed. Therefore the iatrogenic sequence does not proceed beyond the first stage. The point here is that many men may be aware that they are ill, but actively decide not to seek help or socialize this knowledge in order to avoid being labelled as sick. The fixed stereotyping of the male gender role dictates that sickness is seen as an expression of weakness, therefore in the event of illness the stoical, strong and silent bravery of the 'machismo' genre is encouraged by the male gender culture and it is generally not permissible for men to express or display illness as an idiom of distress. This high threshold level for seeking professional help can be counter productive to health (Helman 1994), in that men may ignore a serious condition and seek help too late or may 'play down' the symptoms, causing the doctor to underestimate the seriousness of the problem.

An aspect of the male gender culture that tends to be protective of health rather than pathogenic is the drive to achieve and maintain physical fitness and to transform the appearance of one's body as an expression of self-identity. Growing numbers of both men and women are becoming concerned with body image and self-presentation, so much so that Turner (1992) has introduced the term 'somatic society' to describe the cultural preoccupation with the physical body. This trend is reflected in the establishment of an increasing number of gymnasiums and hotel-based health clubs offering general fitness training and weight lifting. Also, the appearance of magazines such as *Men's Health* that, as the title suggests, concentrate exclusively on men's health and fitness indicates the increase in interest within popular culture of the physical body trend.

Such magazines feature many interesting topics that are beneficial and helpful in that they are health promotional and educational yet the glossy imagery of muscularity encourages a 'cult of physicality' as the dominant conceptualization of masculinity. For those with the potential physique for such a transformation, this may encourage an unprecedented amount of attention to their physical image, whereas those without such potential may be discouraged by a 'spoiled identity' (Goffman 1969).

Shilling (1993) uses the term 'body project' to describe the form of behaviour where the body is considered to be a project to be worked at in order to accomplish optimum health and desirable self-presentation. Many individuals treating their body as a project undertake responsibility for their body and engage in strict self-care regimes. However, this is not to say that all men following a body project regime are well and healthy; for many men following a 'cult of physicality', a high-protein diet that may be considered to be a requirement is often high in animal fats. Also, men's behaviour regarding other health-compromising factors such as alcohol consumption and professional health care avoidance may be evident. Phil Hilton, the editor of *Men's Health*, gives an example of such a paradox in that his magazine, as part of National Men's Health week, surveyed its readers to find that a quarter of them are not registered with a doctor (Hilton 1997). It is perhaps reasonable to argue that men are more influenced to work at their physical shape and appearance with the image of the 'real man' in mind, rather than considering their health from a more holistic perspective.

POSTMODERN MAN

As the male social gender role has evolved from the traditional role to the modern role in order to fulfil the needs of a dynamic and shifting culture, so the postmodern male social gender role ('new man') has now emerged to fulfil the needs of what Giddens (1991) refers to as 'high modernity', that is, the radicalization of modern social trends in late 20th century society. The source of this change is primarily the impact of feminism (Pleck 1976, Harris 1995) on the role and status of women and their cultural interrelatedness with men. Specifically, feminism has shifted the status of women in respect to men from traditional dependence through modern interdependence to the independence and equality of high modernity. This change requires male acceptance of women as peers in the workplace and in the home. In this respect the equal division of domestic power, domestic work and childrearing has led to a social gender 'role shift' where men undertake an equal share or, in some cases, the majority of household tasks and child care responsibilities, whereas women may choose to leave the home to go to work as the equal or sole income provider.

In terms of health and health care, the postmodern male role can be seen as both protective and pathogenic. As the role concerns a considerable involvement with the home and children it is reasonable to assume that many men with domestic responsibility will undertake the role of health care provider for the family and will in that sense be protective of health. However, the postmodern male role represents a major role departure from male gender culture expectation and in terms of personal health may, because of this departure, be at best problematic and at worst significantly pathogenic. The conflicting expectation within the role is essentially a contradiction of masculine identity and this may give rise to the phenomenon termed by Pleck (1976) 'sex [i.e. gender] role strain' and later by Harris (1995) 'gender role stress'. In response to such role stress, problems diverse in nature may result in various idioms of distress, ranging from personality changes such as anger and impatience to physical symptoms such as idiopathic chest or back pain. Further to this, some men affected by anxiety derived from conflicting role expectations may develop various degrees of 'compensatory masculinity' (Harrison 1978) which can, if the behaviour is strongly motivated by the need to demonstrate and prove the right to masculine status, become alarmingly risk taking and destructive.

CONCLUSION

To conclude, it is not my intention to present a sociocultural model or framework designed to manage and promote men's health. I will, however, venture to put forward four pointers for consideration.

First, although it is clear that men's health is mediated by sociocultural factors such as lifestyle choices, it has to be recognized that the aetiology of illness and disease is a multifactorial process in that there are many variables along the so-called 'chain of causality'. Therefore, it would be folly to consider sociocultural factors in isolation from the vitally important anatophysiobiochemical factors. Conversely, concentration on the latter at the expense of the former may be just as devastating.

Second, as a 'sociocultural' caveat, it is worth remembering that cultures are never homogeneous. Therefore one should beware of broad generalizations pertaining to the beliefs and behaviours of human groups. All persons belonging to a cultural group are individuals and often do not behave in a fixed stereotypical fashion.

Third, if it is accepted that male gender role behaviour is a sociocultural construction and that all human behaviour is learnt, then it follows that behaviour can be unlearnt or reconstructed. In other words, in an individual whose lifestyle is clearly pathogenic, the negative behaviours may be reconstructed or modified in collaboration with the individual. An example of this approach is the adoption of the body project concept (with ownership held by the individual) in the rehabilitation and post-rehabilitation phases of myocardial infarction recovery.

Finally, and in respect to the previous point, all modifications of behaviour ought to be balanced with cultural awareness and sensitivity. Drastic reconstruction may be counterproductive, an example being the modification of a type A behaviour pattern that may, somewhat paradoxically, cause the individual to perform to a less satisfactory level at work. The best approach therefore is perhaps a balanced modification in all things.

REFERENCES

Aitchison J 1976 The articulate mammal: an introduction to psycholinguistics. Hutchinson, London

Bernstein B 1971 Class, codes and control. Vol. 1. Routledge and Kegan Paul, London

Brannon L 1996 Gender: psychological perspectives. Allyn and Bacon, Needham Heights, Mass

Brannon R 1976 The male sex role: our culture's blueprint of manhood and what it's done for us lately. In David D S, Brannon R (eds) The forty-nine percent majority. Addison-Wesley, Reading, Mass pp. 1–45

Carrithers M 1992 Why humans have cultures. Oxford University Press, Oxford

Dawkins R 1997 Climbing Mount Improbable. Penguin, Harmondsworth

Douglas M 1973 Natural symbols, 2nd edn. Barrie and Jenkins, London

Frankenburg R 1980 Medical anthropology and development: a theoretical perspective. Social Science and Medicine 14B: 197–207

Friedman M, Rosenman P H 1959 Association of specific overt behavior pattern with blood and cardiovascular findings. Journal of the American Medical Association 169: 1286–1296

Giddens A 1989 Sociology. Polity Press, Cambridge

Giddens A 1991 Modernity and Self-Identity. Polity Press, Cambridge

Goffman I 1969 Stigma: notes on the management of spoiled identity. Penguin, Harmondsworth

Grayson D 1990 Donner Party deaths: a demographic assessment. Journal of Anthropological Research 46 (3): 223–242

Green J 1987 Patterns of eating in normal men and women. Psychology: A Quarterly Journal of Human Behaviour 24 (4): 1–14

Harris I M 1995 Messages men hear: constructing masculinities. Taylor and Francis, London

Harrison J 1978 Warning: the male sex role may be dangerous to your health. Journal of Social Issues 34 (1): 65–85

Helman C G 1994 Culture, health and illness, 3rd edn. Butterworth-Heinemann, Oxford

Herzfeld M 1985 The poetics of manhood: contest and identity in a creton mountain village. Princeton University Press, Princeton

Hilton P 1997 So long, John. The Guardian, health supplement, June 10, p. 15

Hodin J P 1972 Edvard Munch. Thames and Hudson, London

Horrocks R 1995 Male myths and icons: masculinity in popular culture. Macmillan, London

Lewin M 1984 Rather worse than folly? Psychology measures femininity and masculinity. In: Lewin M (ed) In the shadow of the past: psychology portrays the sexes. Columbia University Press, New York

Marmet M G, Syme S L 1976 Acculturation and coronary heart disease in Japanese Americans. American Journal of Epidemiology 104: 225–247

Mauss M 1973 Techniques of the body. Economy and Society 2 (1): 70–88

Mechanic D 1978 Sex, illness, illness behaviour and the use of health services. Social Science and Medicine 12B: 207–214

Pleck J H 1976 The male sex role: definitions, problems, and sources of change. Journal of Social Issues 32 (3): 155–164

Rosenman P H 1978 Role of type A behaviour pattern in the pathogenesis of ischaemic heart disease, and modification for prevention. Advanced Cardiology 25: 35–46

Scheper-Hughes N, Lock M M 1987 The mindful body: a prolegomenon to future work in medical anthropology. Medical Anthropology Quarterly. 1 (1): 6–41

Shilling C 1993 The body and social theory. Sage, London

Shilton H 1996 The pain clinic encounter. MSc dissertation (unpublished). Department of Medical and Social Anthropology, University of Keele, Staffordshire

Turner B S 1992 Regulating bodies: essays in medical sociology. Routledge, London

Waldron I 1978 Type A behaviour pattern and coronary heart disease in men and women. Social Science and Medicine 12B: 167–170

Whitehead M 1988 Inequalities in health: the Black Report and the health divide. Penguin, Harmondsworth

The sexual male

Tony Harrison

INTRODUCTION

The sexual male and male sexuality is a topic worthy of volumes rather than just one chapter. Sexuality and sex are complex areas of the human experience. Definitions of sexuality and sex abound although this author, along with Batcup & Thomas (1994), would suggest that no adequate definition has been reached which can be universally utilized in health care. Barole's (1986) definition gives some indication of the breadth of the topic: 'Genitals are given, what we do with them is a matter of creative invention, how we interpret what we do with them is what we call sexuality'.

The fact that we are discussing only those individuals who have one particular type of genitalia does not make the discussion any less complex. This being the case, it is necessary to structure our examination of the sexual male so as to allow meaningful investigation of some of the more important issues rather than skimpy recounting of them all.

As we are considering the sexual male within the context of health care, one specific framework which suggests itself as a starting point is the WHO definition of sexual health. This states that sexual health is:

- a capacity to enjoy and control sexual and reproductive behaviour in accordance with a social and personal ethic;
- freedom from fear, shame, guilt, false belief and other psychological factors inhibiting sexual response and impairing sexual function;
- freedom from organic disorders, diseases and deficiencies that interfere with sexual and reproductive functions.

While it could be argued that this definition is somewhat idealized, as is the case with other WHO definitions of health, it does at least give us a focus for meaningful discussion. Some issues which would be pertinent to this chapter are discussed elsewhere in this text, including fertility problems, genetics and cultural contexts of behaviour. Here, we will look at some of the other issues, using the WHO definition as a guide.

A CAPACITY TO ENJOY AND CONTROL SEXUAL AND REPRODUCTIVE BEHAVIOUR IN ACCORDANCE WITH A SOCIAL AND PERSONAL ETHIC

Despite the commonly held belief, sex and its expression is anything but someone's private business. Possibly more than any other area of human activity, sexual behaviour is controlled, demarcated and defined by the social and cultural norms of the society in which the individual lives. A capacity to enjoy sexual activity therefore requires either concealment from socially adverse reactions or the expression of sexuality within the socially acceptable mores of the time. It may seem strange, but it could be argued and supported by nearly all readers, at least anecdotally, that some men do have less than enjoyable sex lives. Behaviourists would suggest that a behaviour that is not enjoyable is not repeated but this may not be the case in the human male where social convention (e.g. marriage) may override that lack of enjoyment. Many rationales have been given for why men may have less than adequate sex lives, these being the nature and quality of the relationship in question, social pressure, physical problems, etc., and we will return to these in due course. Simplistic as it may seem, however, a starting point must be, at least under this definition, that an unhappy sex life is also an unhealthy one and the cause of that dissatisfaction needs to be identified and addressed.

Spence (1991), when discussing cognitive-behavioural approaches to sexual therapy, notes that:

Failure to consider the interactional aspects of sexual behaviour, the couple's general relationship and the influences of family and sociocultural environment is likely to result in failure to tackle some important sources of influence over sexual functioning. (p. 115)

Whilst it should be remembered that this quote is from the perspective of a therapist talking about their speciality, it nevertheless illustrates that such considerations should be aired when couples say they are having difficulties. It may be that the relationship difficulty is not sufficient to warrant specialist intervention or it could be that the couple would benefit from organizations like Relate or the intervention of counsellors.

There are many potential causes of relationship difficulty, most of them beyond the scope of this chapter. However, many relationship problems stem from problems of maleness or, indeed, male views of femininity.

The definition we are working from also raises the issue of control.

Issues of control feature in many male-related sexual problems, with rape as an extreme example. More commonly, Stainer-Smith (1993) notes that 'The matter of who is in control colours many psychosexual problems' (p. 87). While discussing contraception and men, he further notes that it may be a contributory factor in impotence of all types and that many men have a stereotype of maleness based around aggression and man as the 'hunter'. It is conceivable that those who hold such stereotypes may actually *need* to feel a sense of control or dominance in order to function sexually. Whether or not this need constitutes a right or is in any way compatible with their partner's desires seems to be at the heart of whether such feelings could be deemed healthy. The problem for men, and one identified by many of Stainer-Smith's sample, is actually talking about such feelings with anyone of either sex.

It could be assumed that the political incorrectness of notions of sexual power inequalities has not helped this scenario. As with many things, perhaps the issue is not one of inequality but of degree. Power taken to extremes and out of context can move from the titillatingly healthy to the abusive and patently unhealthy and even dangerous. Ideas of social and personal ethics become a problem here. What is the social norm for men in relation to sexual activity and expression? If the social norm is constituted within the majority view then, given the power of maleness in society, the accepted view of appropriate male sexual expression is the hunter, the breadwinner, the heterosexual and the stud. This view has been repeatedly challenged by feminists as being an unhealthy relationship base, but this challenge has come from the middle-class intelligentsia rather than the masses, so who actually decides the subtleties of the social norm?

The social norm in most cases constrains or patterns the personal ethic enshrined within the WHO definition, the implications being that such personal ethics are culturally defined. But if this is the case, where does that place us in relation to, say, female circumcision? This act, male orientated but inflicted on women, certainly has a cultural heritage but is now considered by many as an unacceptable violation of women. Perhaps, therefore, we could speculate that sexual mores are culturally attenuated by the immediate culture and can be further affected by ideologies, which are not specific to one culture alone. Such ideologies frequently arise from the developed world and predominantly from the work of feminists within that world. The danger here is obviously of cultural and moral imperialism. Given that all morality is relative to some framework, who is the final arbiter of what is acceptable and therefore considered healthy in terms of men's sexual approaches? We are taken from the international moral discussion, down to individual cultures and finally back to the agreed moral framework of the couple/individual (in that order, the notion of a relationship implying compatibility, ideally).

The complexity of defining what is *right* and then extrapolating from that to what is *healthy* is obvious and likely to make the ethicist wince, especially as we are dealing with sex. However, practitioners in care professions do need some yardstick by which an approach to sexual health can be made. 'Whatever the client feels is right for them' would seem a dubious stance and one fraught with difficulties. What, then, can we use to measure men's sexual behaviour and desires in order to gain some view of potential health (providing, of course, that we have sorted out our own sexual baggage and can be reasonably sure that we are not projecting moral judgements from within our own frameworks onto our clients). In their definition of sexual health, some authors have added the addendum that activities which are neither abusive, exploitative or oppressive (Few 1994), i.e. which do no harm to others and, less clearly perhaps, to the self, can at some level be defined as being sexually healthy. However, this approach also raises problems as that which is not harmful is not necessarily good.

While less than ideal (not necessarily denoting that which is good and healthy), the 'no harm' principle is a useable benchmark, albeit one which involves the convoluted definitions and predictions of harm. The sexual activities that cause harm to others are often linked to control, returning to our obvious and earlier example of men who rape. Less clear are those sexual activities that actually do harm to the individual. The man whose sexual desires extend to suffocation fantasies and who undertakes such activities alone can be at great risk but is actually doing no harm to himself, whereas to undertake such activities with another person who is also excited by the same thing may be eminently more healthy and fulfilling.

Control of conception can also be a control facet for men. As Christopher (1993) points out, men may not use contraception because of 'an unconscious wish to control or limit the partner's sexual activity' (p. 12). Arguably, the reverse could also be true with the man wishing to maintain a certain level of commitment associated with not having children. The mutual decisions of birth control can and should be equitable but men are more inclined to expect women to undertake conception control. Recent concerns about non-barrier methods of birth control linked with a greater empowerment of women has led to women rejecting other forms of conception control. Roberts (1993) notes female clients suggesting that men should now arrange contraception via condom use so that the woman can return to a natural rhythm of her body or avoid health concerns related to her current form of contraception. This Roberts calls: 'Now it's your turn' (p. 23).

Goodrich et al (1994) note that the UK condom market is worth £45 million with 150 million condoms sold per annum. This gives us some idea of the prevalence of condom purchase but it is also important to note that not all condoms sold are used for their designed purpose. The Durex

Report (London Rubber Company 1993) notes that the chemist is the preferred purchase point for women, that couples prefer supermarkets and that vending machine sales are almost all to men. The structured family planning services amount for only 7% of condom distribution. These data indicate that men rarely use family planning clinics, which would seem a great pity as much expertise is available on a range of sexual matters. Such clinics should perhaps investigate how they could improve their service to men. Men prefer the anonymity of self-purchase and, of course, there are plenty of condoms about.

However, to contribute to a sexually healthy life, condoms must be available, appreciated, obtained, stored correctly, used correctly and disposed of correctly. This may seem self-evident but given that men have relied heavily on their female partners for contraception in the past, there is now a whole generation of men for whom condom use may be somewhat strange. Failing to advise men on what may seem obvious can be a mistake. Condoms not only affect the health of men in relation to partnership matters or issues of conception but also help prevent communicable diseases, a point to which we will return later.

The availability of the male pill may significantly affect men's acceptance of their role in conception control but it may well take some time to catch on.

FREEDOM FROM FEAR, SHAME, GUILT, FALSE BELIEF AND OTHER PSYCHOLOGICAL FACTORS INHIBITING SEXUAL RESPONSE AND IMPAIRING SEXUAL FUNCTION

Sexual health for either gender is to some extent dependent not only on self-discovery of sexuality and self-definition and personal acceptance but also on social acceptance (some of the ground we have already covered). In terms of 'fear, shame and guilt', we must take a more pragmatic approach and look at what societies actually sanction and, importantly, what they do not.

Many researchers have tried to ascertain what men and women actually do in relation to sex, notably Kinsey's (1948) report on American male sexual behaviour which was the forerunner of many others. Most mass observation research sought to gain data not only about sexual acts but also people's attitudes to those acts. Obviously, social attitudes change and Kinsey's work is now dated but more recent research allows us to look at some aspects of male sexuality and the reaction of either gender to them. These studies may assist us in identifying aspects that current society sees as shameful and considering what the implication of this is.

The Janus Report on Sexual Behavior (1993) detailed the views of a large sample of Americans on specific sexual acts as to whether they could be considered 'normal' or 'deviant'. As a whole sample (1344 men and 1406 women responding to this question), 95% of males and females thought their sexual practices completely normal. The 'normal' acts which were discussed included the following.

Oral sex	88% male	87% female (p. 89)
Talking dirty	58% male	57% female (p. 90)
Anal sex	29% male	24% female (p. 91)

The above percentages are for those respondents who considered the acts in question either 'very normal' or 'all right'. Those behaviours which the authors classified as deviant (in some manner) were as follows, the percentages representing the same agreement (i.e. very normal/all right).

Sadomasochism	8% male	5% female (p. 114)
Crossdressing	8% male	5% female (p. 120)
Fetishes	22% male	18% female (p. 122)
Golden showers (urine and sex)	6% male	3% female (p. 125)
Brown showers (faeces and sex)	3% male	1% female (p. 126)
Necrophilia	1% male	0% female (p. 127)

These figures by no means represent a summary of what is an extensive report but are used to support our current discussion. The notable thing in relation to 'normality' is the remarkable agreement between men and women, with similar numbers of men and women considering such acts 'normal' as a majority of the sample. The deviant category also shows similar agreement between men and women and the majority agreement that the acts in question are by and large less than normal and so less than acceptable. This, of course, does not necessarily imply that people in the sample had never performed such acts but that the answers they gave reflected what they perceived to be acceptable. A fair extrapolation from this would be that the latter category indicates a whole arena of sexual activity whose participants could expect social sanction and possibly, as a result, some sense of guilt.

Having suggested that these sexual activities (arguably common to both genders to some degree) may attract shame, what is the usefulness of knowing this? For practitioners who wish to undertake sexual health promotion with men, it is vital to be aware of what a society may view as 'normal' and 'deviant' as this will dictate not only the degree of subtlety needed in approaching the subject and the technique used but also the view of the man concerned about his own activity. Having defined what is socially acceptable, that must be translated into acceptability with men and their partners on an individual basis. No judgement here is made about the 'rightness' and therefore health of any of the acts; such acts are essentially morally neutral and so must be examined within the context of the individual and couple situation. It must be noted, however, that some of these acts do carry a risk of infection. Brown showers, for example, can transmit hepatitis, gastric infection, worms, etc. and it is important that practitioners advising men in relation to these activities do not only concentrate on fostering healthy relationships and a positive self-image but must also address physical health matters as they pertain to the act in question. In the example given, a man who wishes to indulge in this act needs advice on hepatitis vaccination, noting signs of infection in others and himself, barrier protection, etc.

Homosexuality would seem an easily accessible example of health problems which may arise from fear, shame and guilt instilled in individuals due to societal disapproval. Homosexuality has been both decriminalized (for consenting adults over the age of 18) and demedicalized in this country for some time and so arguably should no longer be viewed as a health problem. However, problems still arise in relation to society's view of homosexuality and so the adjustment of homosexual individuals to their orientation. HIV/AIDS has highlighted the health needs of gay men in a wide range of contexts, because it has affected this group disproportionately.

Taylor & Robertson (1994), in their paper on the health needs of gay men, noted those needs under three headings: 'identity, sexual health and bereavement'. Only the middle category had a predominantly physiological bent; the majority of health needs were related to societal acceptance or approbation, lack of which contributed to adjustment problems, abnormal grief processes, etc. It becomes evident that many health problems related to homosexuality (HIV aside) are in fact social acceptance problems. Stanley (1995), discussing a mass observation study, found that on the whole her respondents significantly either did not understand what homosexuality was and/or disapproved or were revolted by homosexuality.

Gay men's health, then, would be helped by professionals working towards changing societal views, for example by supporting age of consent debates and the repeal of discriminatory legislation while also working with the gay individual to find an equilibrium which allows them to function within some self-definition of health.

Claiming that such issues should be considered under the heading of sexual health may in itself be discriminatory. Many members of society, regardless of sexual orientation or gender, suffer aberrant grief processes; whether those with alternative sexual orientations should have theirs classified as a problem of sexual health because it relates to their acceptance as sexual beings seems to be a point worthy of debate. Grief problems are grief problems regardless of cause; HIV is a multisystem or immunological condition which can be transmitted via sexual intercourse but it is not per se a sexual disorder. Categorization, it would seem, can also be a problem. For the most significant insight on gay men's sexual activity, readers are directed to the work of Project Sigma, whose 'Kinsey' style mass surveys have illuminated the life of the gay/bisexual male (Davies et al 1993).

However, to return to an earlier point, some sexual activities are neither socially acceptable nor within the remit of 'doing no harm' and as such are not seen as healthy options for men by even the most liberal-minded individual. Examples would include paedophilia, necrophilia, rape, etc. Statistical and anecdotal figures gained from workers in the child protection and rape crisis fields would indicate that these sexual activities are predominantly (though not exclusively) perpetrated by men (Reason 1998, p. 150).

Such a gender bias in itself may indicate some significant differences between the sexual male and the sexual female. Claims have been made about the different view of the sexual act and sex in general in relation to gender; in particular, that women view sex within an intimate relationship and promote its tenderness, significance and link to the emotional, while men can view sex as an act in itself not necessarily linked in any way to emotional commitment. This almost bimodal distribution of views between the female 'subjective' and the male 'objective' is linked further to the attributes displayed by either gender in other areas, such as arts and sciences, etc., with the same bias becoming evident. Mass generalizations have occurred in the name of gender and this author would acknowledge that to a great degree we are talking about broad brush strokes. However, the brush strokes in some arguments are so broad on occasion that they must have significance. No one would claim that the objectification of another person for sexual gratification, as in the case of rape, could ever be deemed 'healthy'. However, where do you draw the line? And how dangerous an occupation is line drawing? Such objectification occurs within relationships and some fantasies about rape. This serves to highlight the complexity of the issues when professionals must view the individual man and work with him to a model of health which might include some objectification or some submission/rape fantasies but only to a degree that would be deemed healthy and do no harm. However, this causes us more problems. 'Degrees' of fantasy are difficult to achieve in that artificially applied limits do not exist in the erotic imagination and so the danger arises that fantasies can be created as unhealthy reality or, conversely, that they can remain as healthy fantasy ameliorated by the real world. The abstraction of defining and dealing with men's internal images and behaviours relating to sex and sexuality in order to promote health is much simplified when we look at the final section of the WHO definition.

FREEDOM FROM ORGANIC DISORDERS, DISEASES AND DEFICIENCIES THAT INTERFERE WITH SEXUAL AND REPRODUCTIVE FUNCTIONS

Organic disorders and deficiencies can be grouped under several headings and in several ways. Some, such as those pertaining to impotence, have been dealt with elsewhere in this text. Organic disorders which are generic rather than genital in origin can affect men's sexual desire and ability and their quality of life. Examples of such diseases are commonplace and, indeed, men presenting with problems of sexual function should always have such areas explored first in order to deal with what may be more easily rectified problems. Curtis et al (1995) note that sexual history taking is a definite skill but that it should provide the opportunity for health promotion in all clients. This author's experience is that sexual history taking per se is often better parcelled in an overall assessment which addresses sexuality, sex and function within the broader remit of health as a whole. Within nursing practice, which has several models which claim to address the holistic assessment of clients, this particular topic is often avoided by practitioners because they rather than the client are uncomfortable with it. As previously noted, this misses many opportunities for promoting sexual health in either gender. Further, while such 'holistic assessments' tend to supply large quantities of information, particularly about clients' medical problems, the correlation between such data and potential sexual sequelae is frequently not made and so clients may plod along with silent worries about their function or desire because the practitioner does not anticipate the problem. To give an example, the client taking hypotensive drugs may have erectile difficulties which may concern him. Had such difficulties been anticipated by either the prescribing medical officer or relevant nurse, much anxiety could have been alleviated and indeed an opportunity to discuss any other sexual worries gained.

The correlation between chronic ill health and loss of sexual function/desire/health is also often forgotten although the effects of change of body image resulting from, for example, mutilating surgery are more frequently addressed. Theory abounds in these areas and the problem may therefore be application rather than actual knowledge.

While the effects of generic disease on sexual function and desire are noted, some disorders are specifically related to the genital tract, the so-called sexually transmitted diseases (STDs). Some sexually transmitted diseases acquired via sexual activity have effects which are not primarily sexual in nature; these would include generic diseases such as human immune deficiency virus (HIV) and hepatitis (A,B,C). Despite the predicted 'heterosexual epidemic' of HIV (Lancet 1993), only 13% of recorded HIV cases in 1993 were ascribed to sexual activity between males and females. HIV does affect men disproportionately but predominantly gay men who acquire the virus through sexual activity or male drug misusers who acquire the infection through sharing equipment and/or sex. Seventy-five percent of drug misusers notified to the Home Office in 1993 were men (Home Office 1994). Some have suggested that this indicates a greater tendency to addictive behaviour in men, although this author believes that fewer women drug users register for treatment because they are concerned about how they will be viewed as mothers should it be known that they are drug users.

HIV is a clear example of a disease which is frequently put under the heading of sexual health and frequently treated within STD clinics but which is actually a systemic immunosuppressive disorder. This being the case, it is more suited to the specialism of immunology than sexual medicine; the same could apply to hepatitis.

However, the same is not true of what might be called the 'true' venereal diseases which can be classified according to type.

Bacterial infections
- Gonorrhoea
- Syphilis
- Chlamydia

Protozoal infections
- Trichomoniasis

Fungal infections
- Candidiasis

Viral infections
- Human papilloma virus

Arthropod infestations
- *Phthirus pubis* (the crab louse)

This does not represent all infections and problems seen in genitourinary medicine but gives us a range of examples to examine the impact of these conditions on the male population (and, by extension, on the female population). Dr Johnson argued that there were two types of knowledge: the knowledge he kept in his head and the knowledge he kept in his library. The exact details of any given STD (of which there are many) come under the heading of library knowledge for most professionals, given that individual disorders can be looked up as required.

The DoH figures (1994) for the decade from 1983 to 1993 show a significant rise in the number of diagnosed wart virus and herpes infections, a steady upward trend in candidiasis and gonorrhoea and a general decline in non-specific genitourinary infections (NSGI). Such figures are useful in indicating trends of infection, but it must be borne in mind that they represent only those who attend for diagnosis (and, indeed, return for their result) and not the totality of the infection pool. The same data source differentiates attendance rates for STDs in 1993 in England by gender as shown in Box 4.1.

Box 4.1

• Herpes	Female 12 749	Male 11 602
• Genital warts	Female 35 150	Male 49 450
• Syphilis	Female 464	Male 848
• Gonorrhoea	Female 5539	Male 8744
• NSGI	Female 41 922	Male 65 994
• Candidiasis	Female 51 618	Male 9104
• Trichomoniasis	Female 5472	Male 371

Some of the discrepancies obvious in these figures relate to the symptom presentation of individual STDs. Candidiasis is more notable and difficult for women and so more women present for treatment than men, whereas genital warts may be more obvious on the penile area than around the vagina and so more men present for treatment of those.

Overall, it would appear that women present for treatment more than men. This could be an indication that men are less concerned about their health, that more men have symptomless presentations or that women are more aware of their own health deficits in general. Fogel (1995, p. 207) notes that much STD research and discourse considers women as 'vectors of transmission' and/or focuses on their reproductive capabilities. It could be argued that this attitude sits well with the predominant male/female balance of power; seeing women as infectors of men is an archetypally patriarchal approach. This author has often heard men talking about 'being given' a venereal disease (with the obvious overtones of a malicious present) and seldom heard any client with a venereal disease discuss having been to 'collect' it. The language itself seems to confirm the male as victim and predominantly a victim whose involvement was negligible. Despite this, Fogel cites authors who, in various ways, indicate that most STDs show a 'biological sexism' (Hatcher et al 1994), with women suffering a disproportionate amount of severe complications of STDs, including sterility, problem pregnancies, pelvic inflammatory disease, etc., in comparison with men.

Impotence

While impotence has been discussed in other parts of this text, it is perhaps pertinent here to reflect on the current debate raised by the drug Viagra. The degree of male physical dysfunction implied by the frenzied reaction to this new drug is vast. It is amazing that a society which has such a male view of virility could quietly accept the huge numbers of men clamouring for it, even taking into account that many of them have bought the myth that Viagra enhances *adequate* performance (which it does not). While the large numbers claiming physical dysfunction could, in part, reflect men's erroneous views of what normal function actually is, we are still left with many who are claiming, by self-definition, sexual ill health.

CONCLUSION

Having touched on some disparate aspects of male sexual health and ill health using the WHO guide, we are still brought back to the central essential questions. What is sexual health for men? Why its sudden resurgence as a topic and what is its importance?

Part of the reason is related to the women's health movement. Women's sexual and general health has been a significant part of gender-based health care for some time and undoubtedly owes much of its renaissance to the feminist movements of the 1960s and 1970s. But no equivalent male political movement has existed in the UK so why has men's sexual health arisen as an area of concern in relation to similar concerns for women now enshrined in service provision and care? There may be three possibilities.

Undoubtedly, the advent of HIV and AIDS and the subsequent panic engendered more interest in the risks of genital sex than any preceding campaigns on the issues of sexually transmitted diseases. Seemingly overnight, sex inherited risks which, if existing before, had been obliterated by the advent of antibiotic treatment. Sexual health was now in many minds synonymous with *not* acquiring a fatal disease. It became the avoidance of disease (normally with a focus on condom wearing), a definition of health which most health care professionals would see as too limiting and based on fear, not the best motivator for long-lasting health behaviour change. However, at least for a while, the issue was prominent, which arguably allowed other sexual health issues to see the light of day but it is debatable whether the public and indeed the professionals ever saw sexual health as anything more than merely the absence of disease.

Second, class and fashion seem to have played a part. The new man of the 1980s or, to be more accurate, the new middle-class white affluent male of the 1980s, seemed to be demanding a health focus of his own and this was frequently sexually orientated. The new journal for men in the UK, called *Men's Health*, has seen its circulation increase dramatically. This *Cosmo* for men follows, in this author's opinion, the tried and trusted approach of the expensive women's slick mag. Its focus is frequently semi-sexual or actually sexual, dealing with better bodies, greater attractiveness and so on, all with the aid of expensive advertising aimed at the affluent male who proclaims health is his right. This could almost be conceived as market-led health awareness.

Lastly, it could be argued that some men's health initiatives have been based on the 'Why not us?' model, which looks at services for women and says, using its powerful male voice, why not us? This approach seems almost petulant. It is true that many health professionals are now realizing that men's health has been neglected and that as a result we are seeing increases in many male health-related problems. These pioneers have, however, an uphill struggle to give men's health and, in particular, men's sexual health the holistic and effective approach to care which the women's health movement has gained over the years.

The milieu in which men's health arises as a topic is important if the debate on men's health is ever to be about more than its component parts. The holistic model of health which we seek needs to encompass the areas briefly discussed above but also to construct a model of health which brings them all together into an image of the sexually healthy male. Such positive images are neither common nor accessible and if we as health care providers are to carry forward effectively the debate about men's sexual health such images need to be constructed, identified and promulgated.

Feminism and the women's health movement saw the evolution of a *positive womanhood* which gave women some role models of health which they could move towards. No such models have evolved for men. Chauvinism has few positive connotations in anyone's mind and the male bonding habits of our American cousins seem rather strange to the English culture. The rise of the 'lad' culture (with its three constituent parts of booze, sport and sex) hardly, in this author's opinion, provides that positive imaging which would give a focus for male sexual health. The tension between the male view of the sexually healthy male and the female view of the sexually healthy male leads to polarization towards the extremes – the lads and the new men. Given this hypothesis, maybe it is time for those who specialize in health to accept the difficult task of developing a definition of what it actually is.

REFERENCES

Batcup D, Thomas B 1994 Mixing the genders: an ethical dilemma. How nursing theory has dealt with sexuality and gender. Nursing Ethics 1(1): 43–52
Barole M D 1986 Body politic/body pleasured. Frontiers. University of Colorado, Boulder, CO
Christopher E 1993 Unconscious factors in contraceptive care. Understanding ambivalence and poor motivation. In: Montford H, Skrine R (eds) Contraceptive care. Chapman and Hall, London
Curtis H, Hoolaghan T, Jewitt C 1995 Sexual health promotion in general practice. Radcliffe Medical Press, Oxford

Davies P, Hickson F, Keogh P, Weatherburn P 1993 The gay men's sex survey at Pride 93. Project Sigma and Gay Men Fighting AIDS, London

DoH 1994 GUM clinic returns 1993. Summary of information from form KC60. Department of Health, London

Few C 1994 Promoting sexual health. Community Outlook 4(2): 29–31

Fogel C I 1995 Sexually transmitted diseases. McElmurry B J, Parker R S (eds) Annual review of women's health, vol 2. National League for Nursing, New York

Goodrich J, Lang H, Sayers M 1994 Health update 4: sexual health. Health Education Authority, London

Hatcher R A, Trussell J, Stewart F et al 1994 Contraceptive technology, 16th edn. Irvington Publishers, New York

Home Office Research and Statistics Department 1994 Statistics of drug addicts notified to the Home Office 1993. Home Office statistical bulletin 10(94). HMSO, London

Januss S S, Janus C L 1993 The Janus Report on sexual behaviour. John Wiley and Sons Ltd, New York, NY

Kinsey A C, Pameroy W B, Martin C E 1948 Sexual behaviour in the human male. W B Saunders, Philadelphia, PA

Lancet 1993 Editorial. Heterosexual AIDS: pessimism, pandemics and plain hard facts. Lancet 347: 863–864

London Rubber Company 1993 The Durex report 1992. A summary of research into usage of condoms and attitudes towards them. LRC, London

Reason L 1998 Abuse, power and sex. In: Harrison T (ed) Children and sexuality. Perspectives in health care. Baillière Tindall, London

Roberts M 1993 The method and its meaning. In: Montford H, Skrine R (eds) Contraceptive Care. Chapman and Hall, London

Spence S H 1991 Psychosexual therapy: a cognitive-behavioural approach. Chapman and Hall, London

Stainer-Smith A 1993 The man and the method. In: Montford H, Skrine R (eds) Contraceptive care. Chapman and Hall, London

Stanley L 1995 Sex surveyed 1949–1994. From mass observations: Little Kinsey to the National Survey and Hite Report. Taylor and Francis, London

Taylor I, Robertson A 1994 The health needs of gay men: a discussion of the literature and implications for nursing. Journal of Advanced Nursing 20: 560–566

5

Men and fertility

Elizabeth H. E. Pease

INTRODUCTION

Man's fertility cannot be fully assessed as an independent entity, successful conception being dependent on the delicate balance between the potential fertility of both the male and his female partner within a heterosexual relationship. If men in a homosexual relationship wish to father a child then obviously the fertility of the surrogate host is of relevance. In vivo, the only true test of fertility is ultimate conception, with in vitro fertilization (IVF) providing the only definitive laboratory test of true sperm function.

Procreation is assumed to be a basic right of the human species. Biblical references such as 'Be fruitful and multiply upon the earth' (Genesis, Ch. 8, vs. 17) give emphasis to this fact. In the male, fertility is still equated with virility, potency and the 'macho image'. This is clearly exemplified by broadsheet newspapers highlighting medical reports of falling sperm counts with headlines such as 'Goodbye macho man' (Daily Telegraph, November 1992) and 'Why today's man is losing his virility' (The Independent, January 1997). Fatherhood and manhood are seen to be inexorably linked, leading to such bar-room jokes as 'jaffa' or 'firing blanks' directed to the childless azoospermic man, only serving to increase the stigma associated with his infertility. Surprisingly, the man who has chosen 'voluntary infertility' by undergoing a vasectomy seems to be excluded from such banter, according to the views of many patients.

A man's emotional needs must not be forgotten or neglected during the investigation and treatment of infertility. Many couples experiencing infertility talk of their grief about being childless, describing their feelings as those of bereavement with 'no tangible loss on which to focus' (Emery 1995).

The past 50 years have seen an increasing awareness and acceptance of the male aspect of a couple's fertility. No longer does the burden of infertility automatically rest upon the shoulders of the female partner. Society in general now accepts the need for male factor investigations in conjunction with those of his female partner. In past times, even the suggestion of the need for male factor screening was seen as a slight against manhood. Women carried the burden of the infertility problem simply to save face on their partner's behalf amongst their peers. The 'barren wife' was a sad but socially acceptable cause of childlessness.

REASONS FOR INFERTILITY

Statistics reveal that 15% or one in six of all couples experience involuntary infertility (Lipshultz & Howard 1983, Hull et al 1985). In up to 40% of cases there is a relevant male factor related to abnormality in sperm concentration or sperm quality parameters. A semen analysis provides a predictive assessment of potential fertility but the report must be interpreted in the context of accepting that eventual fertilization involves a single sperm (spermatozoon) achieving successful penetration of an egg (oocyte). Men with 'normal sperm counts' (normozoospermia) may not achieve conception whilst their oligozoospermic counterparts (those with reduced sperm count and/or quality parameters) prove successful. Cynics may argue 'paternity' in such cases though the advent of IVF has confirmed fertilization to be possible in such patients within the laboratory.

Variability in an individual man's semen production must also be considered. Perhaps increasing attention should be given to the semen quality of putative fathers attending the antenatal clinic with their partners rather than focusing on that of the infertile man. Conception has negated the need for semen analysis in the former group of men. Such a study may allow us to gain further insight into the many mysteries of spontaneous conception.

There are five areas to explore relevant to male factor infertility.

1. Sperm production – testicular spermatogenesis, male gamete production
2. Internal (in vivo) sperm transport within the male
3. Delivery of sperm to the female genital tract
4. Internal (in vivo) sperm transport within the female genital tract
5. Binding and penetration of the egg (oocyte) by the sperm within the fallopian tube – gamete fusion and fertilization.

Spermatogenesis

The testes can be identified by the seventh week of intrauterine life. They initially develop as intraabdominal organs and only descend into their normal scrotal position by traversing the inguinal canals during the ninth month of gestational life. This journey occurs in response to a temporarily increased production of androgens (male sex hormones) from the hormone-producing testicular interstitial cells. It is therefore not abnormal for premature male infants to be delivered with undescended testicles but full-term infants require careful review. Delayed descent can occur up to 3 months of age but spontaneous descent is extremely unlikely after a boy's first birthday. Thereafter consideration must be given to surgical descent and scrotal fixation (orchidopexy), preferably before the boy's sixth birthday, to reduce the likelihood of impaired future spermatogenesis or increased prevalence of testicular cancer in adult life (Whitaker 1975).

Puberty is heralded by testicular enlargement in response to increased pituitary gland activity, resulting in increased output of circulating follicle-stimulating hormone (FSH) and luteinizing hormone (LH). Eighty percent of the bulk of the mature testicle is made up of sperm-producing tissue – the seminiferous tubules. Maturation and functional activity commence within the sperm-producing cells in response to signals from the support cells (Sertoli cells), dependent upon increased pituitary production of FSH. Luteinizing hormone stimulates the Leydig cells to produce testosterone (male hormone). Sperm production within the seminiferous tubules occurs from the age of 11–13 years in response to FSH secretion. The associated development of the normal male secondary sexual characteristics of puberty, including penile development and the growth of facial and body hair, occurs in response to the increasing circulating testosterone levels.

Testicular size in the postpubertal male gives an indication of the man's potential for sperm production. Testes of small volume (i.e. less than 15 ml) are suggestive of compromised spermatogenesis and of a reduction in seminiferous tubular mass. A solitary but otherwise normal testis is capable of entirely normal sperm production capacity. However, normal secondary sexual characteristics and a normal testosterone level do not always equate with normal testicular size and normal spermatogenesis. Such a man may have seminiferous tubule failure, i.e. arrest of germ cell development with intact Leydig cell activity (hormone production). Clinically he would be infertile and have bilateral small soft testes – primary testicular failure.

Sperm transport within the male

Sperm leave the testis via microscopic tubules (the rete testis) and pass into the epididymis, the first collecting system. The epididymis is a multi-coiled tubular structure divided anatomically into head, body and tail regions, the tail leading directly to the vas deferens. Maturation of the sperm, allowing them to achieve the functional competence necessary for fertilization, occurs during the journey through the epididymis. The vasa deferentia are two narrow tubular structures of some 45 cm linear length in total, leading from the epididymis to the base of the bladder. Here they are joined by the ducts of the seminal vesicles to form the ejaculatory duct which passes behind the prostate gland to become the prostatic urethra and finally the penile urethra.

Internal obstruction

Sperm retrieved by direct aspiration from the epididymis are found to be immature and relatively incapable of fertilization unless utilized in the new assisted conception treatment – intracytoplasmic sperm injection (ICSI) IVF. Congenital abnormalities resulting in the absence of the body or tail of the epididymis or vas deferens or failure of canalization of the vas will result in obstructive azoospermia with possible dilatation of the head of the epididymis. Inappropriate surgery to remove swellings palpable in the epididymis may excise the only sperm reservoir present and result in future sterility at a time when the patient has not given his potential fertility consideration. Congenital failure of canalization of the rete testis will prevent the exit of sperm from the testis. Similarly genital infections, e.g. *Neisseria gonorrhoea*, chlamydia or tuberculosis, may be an acquired form of tubular obstruction, affecting proximally the epididymis and distally the region of the ejaculatory ducts.

Delivery of sperm to the female genital tract

Penile size, unlike testicular volume, is rarely related to impairment of fertility, thereby dispelling the popular myths. Ineffective ejaculation may result from phimosis – tightness or abnormality of the foreskin – or from an acquired stricture of the urethra or urethral meatus. An ectopic position of the urethral meatus (hypospadias or epispadias) may in severe cases prevent adequate intravaginal sperm delivery at ejaculation. Acquired penile deformity secondary to Peyronie's disease may cause penetrative difficulties. Very rare cases of congenital absence of the penis also occur. Phalloplasty (surgical reconstruction of the penis) is occasionally attempted.

Erectile dysfunction

Discussion relating to psychosexual dysfunction is addressed in the appropriate chapter of this text. In summary, normal ejaculation requires:

1. adequate sexual stimulation to produce an erection;
2. orgasm/climax;
3. closure of the valve mechanism at the bladder neck;
4. emission of semen into the prostatic urethra;
5. expulsion of semen into the penile urethra followed by external emission via the external urethral meatus on the glans penis.

The majority of the ejaculate, 70%, is composed of secretions from the seminal vesicles and only 30% is from the prostatic urethra. Hence, a man with a proximal blockage may not exhibit a significant reduction in the volume of his ejaculate although there is a total absence of sperm. Similarly, a small volume ejaculate may be indicative of distal blockage in the region of the ejaculatory ducts.

Retrograde ejaculation (dry orgasm)

Such patients experience a normal climax but because of defective bladder neck closure, expulsion of the ejaculate occurs directly into the bladder rather than the penile urethra. Recognized causes are:

1. neurogenic – spinal cord lesions or neuropathy, e.g. complication of diabetes;
2. iatrogenic – secondary to surgical procedures.

Patients undergoing lumbar sympathectomy for peripheral vascular disease or excessive sweating are likely to experience retrograde ejaculation due to the loss of sympathetic nerve activity on the bladder neck. All patients considering transurethral prostatectomy or bladder neck surgery because of poor urinary flow who might wish to maintain their potential fertility must be advised of the possible postoperative complication of retrograde ejaculation. The nature of the resection may damage the valvular closure mechanism at the bladder neck. Preoperative sperm banking as a precaution to maintain possible future fertility requires discussion. Extraction of viable sperm from postmasturbatory urine samples in proven cases of retrograde ejaculation can yield sperm suitable for assisted conception – intrauterine insemination (IUI) (Scammell et al 1989) or in vitro fertilization (IVF).

Premature or retarded ejaculatory dysfunction may be helped by appropriate psychosexual counselling. Artificial insemination is an alternative option for intractable cases.

Sperm transport within the female genital tract

Ejaculation releases seminal fluid into the vaginal vault. Liquefaction occurs and motile sperm gravitate to the healthy environment of the receptive endocervical mucus present during the immediate preovulatory phase of the female's menstrual cycle. Motile sperm traverse the endocervical canal and gain access to the endometrial (uterine) cavity and finally the fallopian tubes via the internal tubular ostia. Motility of the sperm within the genital tract is dependent upon the sperm's inherent, intact, forward propulsive motion.

Gamete fusion and fertilization

During their passage through the genital tract, discrete changes in sperm motility transform the sperm to aid their eventual potential for fertilization. Fertilization is thought to take place within the ampullary region of the fallopian tube. Specific binding receptor proteins allow the sperm to recognize the egg and increase the affinity of one for the other. Hyperactivated motility develops in the sperm in response to capacitation, allowing the sperm to penetrate the outer membrane of the egg (zona pellucida) successfully. In normal fertilization only a single sperm gains access to the cytoplasm of the egg. Without the presence of millions of additional sperms accompanying it on its journey through the genital tract, it is unable in vivo to acquire its final goal.

DIAGNOSIS OF INFERTILITY

In 1992, the European Society for Human Reproduction and Embryology (ESHRA) defined normal fertility as a couple achieving pregnancy within a 2-year period of regular, unprotected coitus. The World Health Organization (WHO) suggested in 1993 that normal fertility was compatible with conception occurring within a 12-month period of unprotected coitus. Specialists differ as to which of these definitions they adhere to but, in the main, investigations would certainly be recommended after a 12-month period especially if the female partner was reaching her mid-30s (Maroulis 1995).

Primary care assessment

The sympathetic ear of a friendly general practitioner at the man's initial consultation can be of immeasurable help and support to the anxious man worried about his fertility. Mishandling of the patient at this very sensitive stage, when he has just voiced his anxiety, can cause untold future emotional trauma. To treat the male partner simply as a producer of a sperm sample, not to mention dealing with his results through the intermediary of his wife/partner rather than directly with the man himself, is a recipe for disaster. Careful initial history taking is needed, enquiring as to whether the man is suffering with primary or secondary infertility, i.e. has he achieved pregnancy with his present or a previous partner? He may not wish to divulge to his present partner proven fertility with an ex-partner or a past history of venereal disease. Enquiry must be made regarding coital frequency and whether he experiences erectile or ejaculatory difficulties. Attention to past medical and surgical history together with social history covering alcohol and cigarette consumption and drug use completes the necessary preliminary enquiries. A brief clinical examination to confirm normal secondary sexual characteristics and the presence or absence of normal testes is relevant at this stage.

First-line investigations

A semen analysis is a straightforward investigation for the majority of patients. However, cultural and religious objections must be taken into account before assuming that this is acceptable for the patient. According to Islamic teaching, masturbation is not permitted by strict Muslims. Similarly, Roman Catholics strictly adhering to their faith are prevented from producing a masturbatory semen sample, as are Orthodox Jews. Coitus using a non-spermicidal condom (silastic condoms) with subsequent transfer of the ejaculate into an appropriate container may be an acceptable alternative to masturbation for some but, again, not for all. Confirmation of intravaginal ejaculation together with the identification of presence of sperm within the ejaculate can be achieved by sampling the vaginal vault contents plus cervical mucus after coitus, i.e. a postcoital test.

Clear instructions must be given to the patient prior to producing his sperm sample by masturbation to ensure that it has been collected under optimum circumstances, allowing the laboratory to produce a more meaningful report.

1. Abstain from any form of ejaculation for 3–5 days before producing the sample, to maximize the number of sperm present.
2. The sample is to be produced by masturbation and collected directly by the patient into a non-spermicidal wide-mouthed container appropriately labelled with the name and approximate time the sample was produced.
3. The sample is to be delivered to the local andrology laboratory, preferably within 30 minutes, and should be maintained at an ambient temperature (25–40°C) en route to the hospital to maintain sperm quality.

The recent establishment of interlaboratory national external quality assurance schemes (NEQUAS) aims to reduce interlaboratory variations in reported interpretations of semen analyses and to prevent unnecessary repetition of samples on the patient's behalf.

Basic semen analysis reports provide the following information.

1. Volume of the total ejaculate.
2. Colour and consistency.
3. Sperm concentration per ml of the ejaculate.
4. Graded quality of sperm motility.
5. Percentage of sperm with normal morphological characteristics.
6. Presence of agglutination – sperm appearing to stick together rather than having totally independent motility.
7. Presence of fructose – secreted by the seminal vesicles.
8. Presence of pus cells (leucocytes) indicating a possible infection and necessitating bacteriological culture of the sample.

The WHO manual of 1987 classifies the following parameters as equivalent to a normal semen analysis, providing the sample has been examined within 60 minutes of production and the analysis performed at 37°C on a heat-staged microscope after thorough mixing on a roller system.

Time of liquefaction	Within 20 minutes
Volume	2–4 ml
Colour	Grey/yellow
pH	7.2–8.2
Fructose	Present
Sperm concentration	> 20 × 10^6/ml
Sperm morphology	> 30% normal forms
Sperm motility classification	> 25% excellent
	> 25% sluggish
	< 50% non-progressive
	< 50% immotile

If the report suggests 'normal spermatogenesis', the patient can be reassured and investigations commenced on his partner's behalf. Should an abnormal report be received this must be sensitively discussed with the patient and he should be advised to repeat the analysis in 4–6 weeks' time whilst arrangements are made for his onward referral to a urologist with a specific interest in infertility or to a gynaecologist specializing in male infertility.

Specialist referral to a secondary centre

Many district general hospitals now have outpatient clinic services specializing in infertility investigations. Patient groups and medical practitioners alike have long pressed for such facilities to be removed from the general urology or gynaecology outpatient clinics. Infertile patients are not, after all, physically ill but they require time, the ear of an interested and well-informed listener together with surroundings appropriate to allow the divulgence of very personal aspects of their lives together with their partner if they so wish.

Subspecialization within medical practice aims to ensure that the specialist to whom the patient is referred has empathy with him and updated knowledge of possible investigations and treatment options open to the patient. The specialist aims to exclude possible treatable causes of sperm malproduction or obstructive delivery before referring the patient onwards to the regional tertiary referral centre for assisted conception, if appropriate or available.

Financial restraints imposed within the NHS have resulted in a marked regional variation in the availability of such services, some regions placing a higher priority and relevance upon their need than others. Rationing of NHS resources will always be a contentious issue when the cost of infertility treatment is set against the need to fund treatment for patients suffering with cancer or heart disease or the need for intensive care facilities for both children and adults within the individual region.

History review

Sperm production is a continuous process from puberty to death. Unlike the female of the species, there is no specific age barrier to potential male gamete production, men having successfully fathered children in their 80s and 90s. Temporary variation in production is a well-documented occurrence and can follow a severe pyrexial illness such as influenza. Recent statistics (Carlsen et al 1992) have suggested a substantial decline in human semen quality over the past 50 years and a presumed reduction in fertility potential in the older male has resulted in the Human Fertility and Embryology Authority restricting the age of acceptable sperm donors to 55 years.

The duration and nature of the infertility should be noted. Coital frequency, together with a working knowledge of the female partner's fertile period, is vital. Ineffectual coitus, even in this enlightened age, may account for up to 5% of referrals to infertility clinics. Working regularly away from home during his partner's potential fertile period may be a simple 'social' cause of infertility. Similarly, the orthodox Jewish couple may be prevented from having midcycle coitus by adhering to the Law of Nidde if the female has regular short menstrual cycles.

The following conditions must be discussed as relevant features in the man's past medical history.

Chronic debilitating diseases known to be associated with possible infertility

- Diabetes
- Renal disease
- Liver disease
- Thyroid disease
- Tuberculosis
- Ulcerative colitis
- Pyrexial illnesses

Genitourinary problems

- Venereal disease, e.g. gonorrhoea, syphilis, chlamydia, non-specific urethritis (NSU), together with the nature of any treatment
- Urinary symptoms with or without urethral discharge suggesting an inflammatory component
- Orchitis – swelling of one or both testicles especially associated with mumps

Exposure to drugs and radiation

- Cytotoxic drugs
- Sulphasalazine for inflammatory bowel disease
- Steroids, particularly their abuse in body builders
- Alcohol
- Smoking
- 'Recreational' drugs, e.g. marijuana
- Previous X-ray therapy

Occupational exposure

- Excessive heat
- Pesticides or herbicides
- Heavy metals, e.g. lead
- Radioactivity

Respiratory problems

- A history of chronic sinusitis and bronchitis may rarely be associated with sperm motility problems, e.g. Kartagener's syndrome (immotile cilia syndrome with situs invertus) or Young's syndrome (immotile sperm possibly due to secretory malfunction within the epididymis)

Surgical conditions

- Scrotal trauma
- Testicular maldescent or cryptorchidism
- Orchidopexy
- Inguinal hernia repair
- Testicular torsion (twisting of the testicle on its cord causing ischaemia)
- Vasectomy or vasectomy reversal
- Varicocoele
- Prostatic or bladder neck surgery
- Urethral strictures or reconstructive penile surgery because of hypo/epispadias (ectopic urethral meatus)

Erectile dysfunction

Physical examination

The preliminary aim is to confirm that the man is phenotypically male, i.e. of normal height and weight and possessing a normal male bodily configuration. Well-developed secondary sexual characteristics are a prerequisite for potential fertility, i.e. the presence of facial and bodily hair distributed in the pattern of the male escutcheon. The presence of breast tissue (gynaecomastia) in the male indicates possible hormonal imbalance or is suggestive of Kleinfelter's syndrome (the XXY male). Poorly developed secondary sexual characteristics are indicative of an endocrinological component relevant to the man's infertility. Auscultation of the chest and recording of blood pressure complete the assessment of the man's general medical well-being but clinical findings may give rise to the suspicion of Young's or Kartagener's syndromes.

Abdominal examination must include careful inspection and palpation of the inguinal regions to exclude a possible hernia, an ectopically situated testis or the presence of an unsuspected surgical scar. Childhood surgery may have been passed over by anxious parents too embarrassed to discuss its nature with their son as he matures into adult life or too ridden with guilt at having produced a son with cryptorchidism (undescended testicles).

Genital examination

The testes naturally retract if exposed to low temperatures so examination should be undertaken in a warm and relaxed atmosphere. The man should be examined in both the recumbent and standing positions for only in the latter situation will the presence of a varicocoele become apparent. Palpation of a 'bag of worms' within the scrotum is the classic feature suggestive of a varicocoele, i.e. varicose veins developing around the testicular vein as it passes through the spermatic cord.

Gentle scrotal palpation should confirm the presence of two testes, ovoid structures with a firm rubbery consistency positioned in a vertical axis of length 4–5 cm. An orchidometer can be used to confirm the exact testicular dimensions. Small soft testes are indicative of testicular atrophy (primary testicular failure) whereas small hard testes are characteristic of some cases of Klinefelter's syndrome (XXY). Rarely, examination may reveal the presence of an unsuspected testicular mass, i.e. a tumour, unrelated to the infertility, necessitating immediate urological referral for further investigation.

The epididymis lies behind the testicle and is only discretely palpable if enlarged due to infection (epididymitis) or possible outflow obstruction. The vas deferens should be palpable distal to the epididymis within the scrotum as a cord-like structure. Congenital absence of the vas is found in approximately 2% of cases of obstructive azoospermia. Men suffering with cystic fibrosis have an increased likelihood of absent vas deferens (Lancet 1992).

Penile examination should include inspection of the shaft, foreskin and glans penis together with confirming the normal position of the external urethral meatus.

Rectal examination allows palpation of the prostate gland and the seminal vesicles should they be enlarged as a result of inflammation. Prostatic tenderness, with or without enlargement of the gland, may indicate subclinical prostatitis and gentle massage may produce a urethral discharge which can be sent for bacteriological culture and appropriate antibiotic treatment instituted if indicated.

Ultrasound examination of the scrotal contents and transrectal ultrasound can be performed to confirm clinical findings.

Implementation of second-line investigations

Investigations to confirm clinical suspicions are necessary before contemplating onward referral to the tertiary regional centre for assisted conception. The relevance and nature of these investigations must be discussed at length with the patient ensuring that he and his partner fully understand the possible implications of the results. The majority of patients will benefit from a tangible report to allow them to compare their own results with the standard normal range values. Most crave an explanation as to why they have a problem and will pursue every investigation possible to this end. Rarely, a patient will decline investigations, preferring to accept the status quo and simply get on with other aspects of his life. The availability of sensitive infertility counsellors can prove invaluable in helping the man adjust to his infertility and to possible future treatment options at this stage.

Investigations

1. Repeat semen analysis +/– centrifugation to confirm complete azoospermia
2. Antisperm antibodies in seminal plasma
3. Serum FSH and LH
4. Possible chromosome analysis in azoospermic males
5. Testicular biopsy – microscopic confirmation of normal or abnormal testicular histological features
6. Vasography – delineation of the vas using radioopaque dye
7. Examination of postmasturbatory urine if retrograde ejaculation is suspected

Results

Patients fall into three broad categories in terms of their results.

1. Normal – normozoospermic semen analysis with normal FSH level – unexplained male factor infertility
2. Azoospermia
   • with normal FSH – obstructive aetiology
   • with elevated FSH – testicular failure
   • with low FSH – pituitary gonadotrophin release failure
3. Oligozoospermia – low sperm density but normal quality parameters
4. Oligoasthenozoospermia – low sperm density with reduced quality parameters

Group 1 – Normal findings

The reassurance of 'normality' may be sufficient to allow the couple to leave their future chance of conception to nature. Others view the result as a two-edged sword, their initial feelings of relief tempered with an overwhelming sense of despair as to why their problem persists and why the specialist cannot diagnose their condition. Clinicians must be honest with their patients, confirming the present limitations in understanding the complex problem of male infertility. Years must not be wasted prescribing empirical unproven medications before considering assisted reproduction. The two most important predictive factors relevant to successful in vitro fertilization are the duration of the couple's infertility together with the age of the female partner embarking upon treatment. The longer the period of infertility and the older the female partner, the less likely is conception to be achieved (Templeton et al 1996).

Group 2 – Obstructive azoospermia

The feasibility of reconstructive surgery involving the vas deferens and epididymis (vasovasostomy or epididymovasostomy) must be assessed by a urologist experienced in microsurgery techniques.

The finding of an epididymal swelling necessitates referral to the tertiary centre for assessment of suitability for epididymal aspiration, i.e. a diagnostic PESA (percutaneous epididymal sperm aspiration with or without local anaesthetic), or for MESA (microepididymal sperm aspiration – open exploration of the epididymal tubules under general anaesthesia). Should viable immature sperm be retrieved, the possibility of intracytoplasmic injection IVF can be discussed with the couple as a treatment option. With the successful advent of PESA together with ICSI, it is vital that epididymal swellings are not simply excised for cosmetic reasons or for symptoms of pain in a young man attending the urology outpatient clinic without giving thought to his potential long-term fertility. Excision may permanently remove his only chance of sperm retrieval from this obstructed sperm reservoir.

Azoospermia of testicular origin   Absolute confirmation of this diagnosis requires a testicular biopsy. The histological picture will confirm whether or not germ cell activity exists in any of the seminiferous tubules examined. Testicular sperm extraction (TESE), i.e. the washing of spermatocytes from biopsied testicular tissue, is theoretically possible if areas of spermatogenesis are confirmed. These spermatocytes can then be utilized for ICSI IVF. This treatment option is as yet in its infancy within the UK but is a proven treatment option in Brussels (Devroey et al 1994).

Histologically, a testicular biopsy can indicate a likely diagnosis of Klinefelter's syndrome. The relevance of confirmatory chromosomal analysis needs sensitive handling. A definitive diagnosis is a finite confirmation of sterility but the knowledge that they have a genetic make-up including an extra female chromosome may prove hard for patients to come to terms with and cause them undue anxiety. Many andrologists now suggest that a man diagnosed with Klinefelter's syndrome will benefit from long-term testosterone supplements irrespective of his infertility to help maintain normal bone density in later years, an additional positive reason for making the diagnosis.

Permanent infertility must be accepted by this group of patients. However, the man's infertility problem can be bypassed by the couple utilizing sperm donation (DI) to achieve a much wanted planned pregnancy together. This often proves to be a difficult option to consider until the couple have had sufficient time to come to terms with the untreatable diagnosis. Once this has been accepted, donor insemination can be the perfect solution for many couples, allowing them to create a child who, although not genetically related to the male partner, is his legal child and responsibility as per the HFEA guidelines implemented in 1991.

Azoospermia as a result of pituitary gonadotrophin production failure This relatively rare diagnosis is treatable by the administration of exogenous gonadotrophins providing there is adequate testicular tissue capable of a functional response. Up to 50% of such men treated successfully will achieve a pregnancy with their partner.

Group 3 – Oligozoospermia and oligoasthenozoospermia

The aim of treatment within this group of men is to maximize the functional capacity of the seminiferous tubules by, in the main, empirical measures. The maintenance of good general bodily well-being, e.g. weight reduction in the obese male, reduction of alcohol and cigarette consumption together with avoidance of excessive heat to the testicles, is a simple first-line approach. Nature intended the intrascrotal position of the testes to provide an environmental temperature 2°C lower than that of the body to aid normal sperm production activity. Avoidance of regular saunas and lengthy hot baths together with the wearing of loose-fitting boxer shorts will help maintain the naturally reduced testicular temperature.

Inexplicably, some men's testicular tissue appears more sensitive to adverse environmental effects than others, just as not all men who smoke heavily develop lung cancer. As yet, there is no predictive test for susceptible patients so prevention is still better than cure.

Treatment of any suspected low-grade genital infection should involve long-term low-dose antibiotics, e.g. oral doxycycline. Although this may not be of proven efficacy, it is unlikely to cause the patient any deleterious effects.

Varicocoeles occur in 10–15% of the general male population. The incidence is found to rise to 25–40% in men undergoing fertility investigations. Although a much debated question, most urologists would recommend either surgical ligation using open surgery or laparoscopic techniques or embolization of the varicose veins, in the hope of improving sperm quality (WHO 1992). The latter, less invasive treatment option is performed on an outpatient basis and involves guiding a number of inert titanium coils into the testicular vein under radiological control, thereby inducing occlusion. Enthusiasts for this treatment believe that the thermogenic effect of the varicose veins impairs spermatogenesis.

Limitation of sperm motility may be due to the development of anti-sperm antibodies within the seminal plasma. Under normal circumstances sperm are protected within their tubular system from the normal immunological mechanisms of the body. Infection or surgery exposes sperm, which appear to be regarded as foreign bodies, directly to the bloodstream, inducing antisperm antibody production. In the past the treatment of choice has been intermittent high-dose steroid therapy taken by the man in conjunction with the preovulatory phase of his partner's cycle. A significant reduction in antibody titre could be anticipated in approximately 30% of such men. Statistics related to successful conception rates thereafter were poor and because of the possibility of such serious side effects as aseptic necrosis of the head of the femur, this treatment has been superseded by assisted conception – ICSI IVF.

Many men are desperate to try some form of medication to improve their sperm counts. A variety of preparations have been utilized, e.g. clomiphene, mesterolone, testosterone and gonadotrophins. Controlled double-blind trials have shown these drugs to be ineffective in producing sustained improvement in count and/or sperm quality and they are not to be recommended (Hargreave et al 1984).

ASSISTED REPRODUCTION AT A TERTIARY CENTRE

Clinics licensed by the Human Fertilization and Embryology Authority (HFEA) (British Acts of Parliament 1990) can offer treatment utilizing cryopreserved gametes, donated gametes and in vitro fertilization. Each individual unit operates under the strict Code of Practice issued by the HFEA, which gives guidance on how clinics should carry out licensed activities. At all times, the welfare of the child to be created by assisted reproduction techniques must be given priority, in addition to considering the well-being and suitability of the patients wishing to pursue treatment. If a couple wish to proceed with intrauterine insemination (AIH), using the male partner's fresh semen sample, or with GIFT (gamete intrafallopian tube transfer) then they can approach unlicensed clinics as these two forms of treatment fall outside the remit of the HFEA. Embryos are not created outside the body with these techniques nor are gametes stored for future possible use. Hence they are not included in the HFEA guidelines.

AIH with or without stimulation of ovulation is of value to couples with psychosexual difficulties. Providing the man is capable of ejaculation after masturbation, his sample can be delivered to the cervix of his partner using a narrow-gauge syringe either by the infertility clinic staff or by the couple themselves within their home environment after appropriate instruction. AIH can similarly be utilized for paraplegic patients who are able to achieve ejaculation following electrostimulation. Providing motile sperm are retrieved from postmasturbatory urine in men with retrograde ejaculation, AIH can again prove helpful.

Improved conception rates are achieved by performing intrauterine insemination. This involves laboratory preparation of the sample using a 'Pure-Sperm' (swim-up) technique to remove only the viable morphologically normal sperm from the seminal plasma. The sperm are then suspended in 0.4 ml of medium and placed in the fundal region of the uterus at the time of ovulation using a flexible catheter.

Artificial insemination for the oligospermic male is a debatable treatment option. Statistically AIH in such patients, in conjunction with induction of ovulation, is associated with variable success rates. However, if the more successful in vitro fertilization is not an available option for the couple, then AIH could be considered for perhaps a finite course of five or six inseminations.

SEMEN CRYOPRESERVATION

Sperm banking by patients

Successful cryopreservation of sperm has been performed in the UK for some 20 years. Men likely to experience impaired future fertility because of prospective orchidectomy (testicular removal), chemotherapy, radiotherapy or total body irradiation can now deposit semen for storage prior to commencement of the treatment. Within the guidelines of the HFEA such sperm can remain frozen for a period of up to 10 years or longer if the semen is to be used specifically for the man and his partner in due course. It is vital that such men are aware of this option but, more importantly, of the long-term effects of their proposed treatment with respect to their future fertility.

Men anticipating prostatectomy or bladder neck surgery may be offered preoperative semen banking as a back-up should retrograde ejaculation result postoperatively. Following preoperative counselling, men agreeing to vasectomy must accept that the procedure is irreversible. Within the UK it been suggested that perhaps 3% of men having undergone vasectomy will, as a result of a change in the man's social circumstances, request vasectomy reversal (Howard 1982). Patients considering vasectomy may wish to explore the possibility of preoperative semen banking to maintain a chance of potential fertility. Most surgeons would have doubts regarding performing a vasectomy if the man raised major anxieties with respect to his future fertility. Percutaneous epididymal sperm aspiration (PESA) is a new alternative option to vasectomy reversal.

Sperm banking for donation

Within the HFEA guidelines fit, healthy men between the ages of 18 and 55 years can be considered as potential sperm donors. The sperm donor accepts no legal rights for any child conceived whether the donation was made on a known or anonymous basis. The donor's anonymity will be strictly maintained if this was the nature of the donation. All donors are registered within the HFEA and nationally they are limited to the creation of a maximum of 10 children to minimize the chance of half-sibling future relationships. The HFEA were looking towards phasing out payments available to sperm donors (at present up to £15 per sample), wishing to ensure that gamete donation was an altruistic act. Many assisted conception units expressed grave anxieties regarding their future donor supplies if this was imposed and only legitimate incurred expenses were reimbursed after consultation. Present payments will, therefore, continue (HFEA, December 1998).

All potential donors must agree to undergo counselling and a medical examination together with screening for venereal disease. Screening blood tests for hepatitis, HIV (AIDS), syphilis and cytomegalovirus (CMV) are accepted as routine and the donor must attend for follow-up HIV screening 6 months after donation. Only if this second test proves negative may the cryopreserved sperm be thawed and issued to recipient couples.

Rarely, thankfully, a potential donor comes forward willingly only to discover once his semen analysis has been performed that he himself is infertile. This can be a devastating blow for the man and it is obviously important that all donors should be made aware of the possibility before submitting their first sample. Similarly, it is not unknown for a man to attend a sperm bank simply as a means of having a semen analysis performed for his own reassurance, never to return once he has received the report.

IN VITRO FERTILIZATION

In vitro fertilization (IVF) was pioneered by Patrick Steptoe and Robert Edwards in the 1970s, leading to the first successful birth, that of Louise Brown in 1978. The technique had been devised to bypass an obstructive tubal factor on the female's behalf, preventing sperm and egg meeting. More recent ongoing research has proven IVF to be a major breakthrough in the treatment of male factor infertility. For successful conventional IVF, each harvested egg (oocyte) has to be inseminated and cultured within the region of only 100 000 normal sperm. This number of sperm can be retrieved without difficulty from the majority of men with a moderate degree of oligozoospermia.

In cases of severe oligoasthenozoospermia or of failed fertilization with conventional IVF, intracytoplasmic injection (ICSI) of an egg with a single sperm can be performed. This technique is also suitable for the immature sperm aspirated by the PESA/MESA/TESE techniques. ICSI bypasses the need for the sperm to bind and penetrate the egg and can also be effective in cases of total sperm immotility providing the sperm is viable. Although fertilization rates of 80% plus per egg are confirmed with IVF and ICSI

IVF, the overall ultimate pregnancy rate per treatment cycle remains in the region of 20%. The question of fertilization can be answered but whether or not a pregnancy will ensue remains indeterminable.

Anxieties have now surfaced suggesting that ICSI, if successful, may perpetuate male infertility in the next generation. Genetic research has located the gene for spermatogenesis on the long arm of the male Y chromosome with abnormalities being noted in infertile males (Simpson et al 1993). A national survey of ICSI male infertility and microdeletions of the Y chromosome (SIMMY) has been started by Hargreaves et al in Edinburgh to compare the chromosomal pattern of men who successfully father sons after ICSI with that of their sons. Careful scrutiny of the results from this survey will hopefully provide the answer.

Recent papers have reported statistical evidence of a general decline in male sperm production within the past 50 years (Carlsen et al 1992). There is as yet no definite evidence of an associated decline in fertility. This may be explained by the fact that although the total ejaculatory sperm count is reduced, it is still maintained above the lower limit compatible with potential fertility. A report from the Medical Research Council in 1996 showed that men born in the 1970s produced on average 25% fewer sperm than men born in the 1950s. Extrapolating this report to its extreme would suggest that if sperm production declined at the rate of 2% per year then all males born in 60 years time may be infertile. This may, however, be an extreme, statistically flawed view and without knowledge of the cause of the decline in sperm counts, such predictions are mere hypotheses.

Histological evidence of falling sperm production has been provided by Finnish workers (Pajarinen et al 1997). They found a reduction in testicular weight together with a significant drop in sperm production when testicular biopsies were examined from postmortem middle-aged males. The study involved comparing biopsies from men of a similar age distribution dying in 1981 with those a decade later in 1991.

No convincing explanation has yet been put forward for these findings although increasing exposure to oestrogens is the suspected likely hypothesis (Sharpe & Skakkebaek 1993). Intensive farming methods utilizing hormonal supplements have produced an increasing dietary consumption from ingestion of dairy products. Anxieties have been raised retrospectively following foetal exposure to excess oestrogens in the past. In the postwar period women at risk of spontaneous abortion were given stilboestrol until its use was questioned in 1970. Environmental oestrogen production has risen in consequence of society's increasing use of plastics and detergents which contain chemicals which mimic the effects of oestrogen. Once absorbed, the effects of the environmental oestrogen-like substances are prolonged within the body as they take longer to be metabolized in vivo than naturally occurring oestrogens.

European Regulations now require assessment of the effects of occupational exposures upon fertility and the reproductive organs. Renewed efforts to determine answers to these questions has led in 1998 to a proposed UK multicentre investigation of male infertility. The University of Manchester School of Epidemiology in collaboration with the University of Sheffield Department of Obstetrics and Gynaecology aim over the next two years to question 6000 men attending infertility clinics in 10 city centres throughout the UK. Environmental and occupational exposures to chemicals will be studied in conjunction with obtaining possible evidence of intrauterine exposure, infant feeding patterns and dietary intake of phytoestrogens. The result of this major study may confirm or refute today's suspicion that unless the reduction in sperm production is halted, mankind's fertility could be severely compromised as we move into the next millennium.

POSTHUMOUS MAINTENANCE OF MALE FERTILITY

Cryopreservation of semen became regulated by the Human Fertilization and Embryology Authority in 1991. Since that time a man can only legally bank his sperm during his lifetime after completing written consent forms. These forms must stipulate the maximum period of anticipated storage (if this is to be less than the statutory storage period), together with his specific wishes regarding the fate of his gametes should be die or become incapable of varying or revoking his consent. If his sperm is to be utilized by his partner for insemination or IVF, she must be named on the consent form. Without his written consent, his sperm should not be cryopreserved nor can any future use be made of his sperm. In the event of his death the following three options are available:

1. sperm to be allowed to perish;
2. sperm continued in storage for the specific use of his named partner;
3. sperm continued in storage for other purposes – donation and/or research.

Sperm can only legally be maintained in storage after a man's 55th birthday with his consent for specific limited uses.

If a pregnancy is successfully achieved posthumously then in spite of her partner's written agreement to the proposed treatment given during his lifetime, the woman is not permitted to record her deceased partner as father of the child for birth certification purposes. The conception must be accepted in terms of a sperm donation. Similarly, a wife or next-of-kin has no legal ownership of her deceased husband's sperm; it does not form part of his estate. She has no rights to utilize the sperm without his prior consent.

Debate has been reestablished within the House of Lords regarding the rights and wrongs of this legal position. Deeply felt but divergent views have been expressed by lay people, infertility specialists and patients themselves following a recent test case involving a woman's quest to utilize her husband's sperm posthumously without his written consent. The Diane Blood case was, after a High Court hearing, eventually resolved without any change to the present legislation in the United Kingdom. The Human Fertilization and Embryology Authority agreed to the sperm being exported to a clinic in Europe and maintained in storage. The clinic staff advised that they would only consider treatment after detailed counselling and assessment of the patient. (Diane Blood eventually delivered a healthy son in December 1998.) The Authority has stressed that no unit in future should cryopreserve sperm without a man's written consent.

Any change to the present legislation will require careful thought from the point of view of society in general, the patients and the possible children to be conceived. Without adherence to the present legislation, a situation could arise whereby the management of a moribund patient in the accident and emergency department could be complicated by a relative's request for sperm recovery. In such an emergency situation, the implications of future procreation cannot have been considered.

Cynics may argue that money directed towards infertility research and treatment is misspent in view of present world population statistics. Such cynics rarely experience involuntary infertility and fail to appreciate the suffering and heartache that childlessness imposes. Future research will hopefully reveal more answers to the complicated process of spermatogenesis. Nature will always hold the balance and it is unrealistic to envisage a situation of guaranteeing every couple a child. The important factor for the couple is to have allowed them the benefit of investigation and the chance of success with appropriate treatment.

REFERENCES

British Acts of Parliament 1990 Human Fertilisation and Embryology Act. HMSO, London

Carlsen E, Giwercman A, Keiding N, Skakkebaek N E 1992 Evidence for decreasing quality of semen during past 50 years. British Medical Journal 305: 609–613

Devroey P, Liu J, Nagy Z, Tournaye H, Silber S, van Steirteghem A 1994 Normal fertilisation of human oocytes after testicular sperm extraction and intracytoplasmic sperm injection. Fertility and Sterility 62: 639–641

Emery J 1995 Silent suffering. British Medical Journal 311: 1647

Hargreave T B, Kyle K F, Baxby K et al 1984 Randomised trial of mesterolone versus vitamin C for male infertility. British Journal of Urology 56: 740–744

Howard G 1982 Who asks for vasectomy reversal and why? British Medical Journal 285: 490–492

Hull M G F, Glazener C M A, Kelly N J et al 1985 Population study of causes, treatment and outcome of infertility. British Medical Journal 2: 1693–1697

Lancet 1992 Editorial. Congenital bilateral absence of the vas deferens and cystic fibrosis. Lancet 339: 1328–1329

Lipshultz L, Howard S S (eds) 1983 Infertility in the male. Churchill Livingstone, New York

Maroulis G B 1995 Effect of aging on fertility and pregnancy. Endocrinologist 5: 364–370

Pajarinen J, Liappala P, Penttila A, Karhunen P J 1997 Incidence of disorders of spermatogenesis in middle aged Finnish men 1981–1991: 2 necropsy series. British Medical Journal 314: 13–18

Scammell G E, Stedronska-Clark J, Edmonds D K, Hendry W F 1989 Retrograde ejaculation: successful treatment with artificial insemination. British Journal of Urology 63: 198–201

Sharpe R M, Skakkebaek N E 1993 Are oestrogens involved in falling sperm counts and disorders of the male reproductive tract? Lancet 341: 1392–1395

Simpson E, Chandler P, Goulmy E, Ma K, Hargreave T B, Chandley A C 1993 Loss of the azoospermia factor (AZF) on Yq in man is not associated with loss of HYA. Human Molecular Genetics 2: 469–471

Templeton A, Morris J K, Parslow W 1996 Factors that affect outcome of in vitro fertilisation treatment. Lancet 348: 1402–1406

Whitaker R H 1975 Orchidopexy and orchiectomy. British Journal of Hospital Medicine 14: 282–294

WHO 1992 The influence of varicocoele on parameters of fertility in a large group of men presenting to infertility clinics. Fertility and Sterility 57: 1289–1293

FURTHER READING

Hargreave T B 1994 Male Infertility, 2nd edn. Springer-Verlag, London

Mason M C 1993 Male infertility: men talking. Routledge, London

Rowe P J, Hargreave T B, Mellows H J, Comhaire F J 1993 World Health Organization manual for the standardised investigation and diagnosis of the infertile couple. Cambridge University Press, Cambridge

6

Men and parenting

Karen Dignan

INTRODUCTION

The aim of this chapter is to present a view of fatherhood in a holistic way. It is not possible to be exhaustive, but the intention is to present the most important aspects in relation to the role of the father from a social, physical and psychological perspective. It is also important that as health professionals we recognize the value of our role in aiding a healthy transition from the role of husband/partner to that of father.

The importance of men's health has only in fairly recent years attracted any investigation or consideration. The ability to procreate has been afforded even less attention, again until very recent times. The inability to physically conceive a child was seen as predominantly a female problem but it is increasingly recognized that the male reproductive system can also cause problems. The social stigma and psychological distress that male infertility may bring can be traumatizing for the man. He may have to endure insensitive comments from family and friends relating to his prowess as a man.

So where do we begin on the road to becoming a healthy parent?

Becoming a healthy parent

The point at which one becomes a healthy parent is debatable as it relates to many facets of the role of being a parent and of being a healthy individual. It is important to address how society views fatherhood because society's view can often enhance or devalue the role. The change that has occurred in the role of the father, particularly over the past 40 years, has meant that generally men have taken more interest in their partners' pregnancies and have subsequently become more active participants in child care.

Being a healthy parent might start at the child's birth and involve the change in lifestyle practices that might be adopted. Equally, it might start prior to conception as the desire to ensure optimum fitness in order to conceive and achieve a healthy outcome to that conception. This puts being a healthy parent into the physical perspective. There is also the viewpoint that parenting skills and knowledge are passed on through families, which means that parents perpetuate their own parents' behaviour, which may be good or bad. This adds a cultural dimension to the arena. All these factors have an influence upon each other to varying degrees depending on the individual and their circumstances. It is, however, the midwife who is in the prime position of enabling men to become competent and skilled fathers due to the knowledge and skills that she has in relevant spheres. One such area is the part that society plays in structuring the role of fatherhood.

The role of the father has changed considerably over this century from that of being the authoritarian breadwinner to the actively involved participant in baby care. Several factors have been influential in bringing about the changes in paternal involvement and behaviour, the greatest being the change from hierarchical dominance to family collaboration. Where at one time the father as the head of the household made the decisions and the wife and children had to adhere to them, today generally less male dominance and control are exerted and more love and compassion are shown (Bozett & Hanson 1991).

A new man?

Men today do participate more in the running of the household and child care responsibilities than their fathers generally did. The division of household labour is more equal, particularly when the mother returns to employment outside the home. Mackay (1985) does go so far as to suggest that there is no society where there is equal division of child care duties, but that the male is still seen as predominantly the breadwinner responsible for supporting the new family financially. There are, however, social factors which affect how men adopt and adapt to the socially constructed role of father.

Does the socially constructed role of the father exist or is there a more individual and less defined construct of a father? The answer may lie with the phenomenon termed the 'new man'. A new man is one who does not see his role as defined by history or culture. The new man is more sensitive and caring and shows his emotional side without fear of undermining his masculinity (Webb 1994). The change in the fatherhood role may be as much due to altered family circumstances as to anything else. There are increasingly more single parents, either through choice or through separation and divorce. This has led to mothers, in the majority of cases, having custody of the children and fathers having access rights, permitting planned quality time to be spent with their children. One of the influences in the emergence of the new man is the lack of employment prospects for the male and also the fact that his female partner may be in employment that brings greater financial reward. If this is the case then it does appear to make sense that the male should be the prime child care provider. However, in reality the new man is in the minority and not the majority. The father who remains at home and adopts the role of 'house husband' whilst the mother goes out to work may experience isolation and loneliness. The social meeting places where mothers take their children to play, such as play groups and mother and toddler groups, may be uninviting for the father. He may feel, understandably, like the odd one out.

Changing family structure

There has also been a change in the family structure from the extended family to the nuclear family. The extended family unit meant that family traditions and practices relating to childbirth and child rearing were passed down and with that came the support of, predominantly, the female members of the family. This meant that the males were not expected to participate in any of the childbirth or child care practices. The reduced family size, in terms of the number of children couples were having and the improved education of both sexes, has also had a positive effect upon the role of the father. Loss of extended family support has meant that the support has had to come from the man, not only as an active participant in child care and child rearing practices but also in the childbirth process, particularly in terms of being the support person during labour.

Occupation

The healthy aspect of fatherhood is also affected by the type of occupation and the environment in which that occupation is carried out. The employment market has undergone great changes this century, particularly in relation to the male-dominated occupations. The increasing use of technology has had a profound effect upon employment numbers and the type of jobs available. Where at one time a job would be performed by several men, now it may only take one man to operate a machine, with the obvious results that male unemployment has risen. Unemployment in itself brings lack of self-worth and loss of self-esteem which may eventually culminate in clinical depression. This is possibly a factor for the rise in male suicide rates. For those prospective fathers who are fortunate enough to be in paid employment, there may still be fertility risks associated with it.

Employment risk factors associated with the ability to parent a healthy child have undoubtedly improved over this century. Health and safety legislation and the use of protective clothing in certain areas of employment have done much to improve health at work. A man's occupation may be hazardous to his fertility prospects if his work involves exposure to environmental or occupational toxins. There is an abundance of evidence to suggest that exposure to harmful agents does increase the likelihood of spontaneous abortion, preterm delivery, low birth weight infants and congenital abnormalities (Taskinen et al 1989, Savitz et al 1989). A man has some control over this by pursuing a less occupationally hazardous career in order to optimize the chances of having a healthy offspring. However, this is only a minor factor which should be viewed from a wider stance which includes other social and lifestyle issues.

Lifestyle

Lifestyle factors are intrinsically linked in that both may have a profound effect upon holistic health. There are many old sayings, such as 'You are what you eat' or 'Live by the sword and die by the sword', that can be translated into everyday lifestyle issues. Behaviours adopted by the man can have quite profound effects upon the outcome of his partner's pregnancy. Advice on making changes to lifestyle behaviours, such as diet, smoking and alcohol consumption, has always predominantly been directed at the woman as the host for the developing embryo but there is mounting evidence that the lifestyle practices and behaviours of the man can have a damaging effect upon the development and subsequent outcome of that embryo (Bushy & Graner 1990).

Some lifestyle factors cannot be readily changed by the individual, such as the type and condition of the living accommodation or the amount of financial income coming into the household, but there are some quite damaging lifestyle factors which the person can change, should they so wish. The two prime examples are smoking and alcohol consumption. It is totally within the person's control whether or not to indulge and how much to indulge in these harmful drugs. This may seem a harsh stance to adopt as it could be argued that smoking and alcohol are ways of dealing with the stresses of everyday life that some people live with, which in this context means that smoking and alcohol might be viewed as stress relievers.

The effect that alcohol consumption has upon the developing foetus and subsequent infant has been documented by several authors (Robarts 1989, Hyssala et al 1992, Kuller 1994), but the amount of alcohol which may be safely consumed is still uncertain. This has invariably related to the alcohol intake of the female. However, it is now recognized (Summers & Price 1993) that alcohol consumption by the male may affect not only his ability to perform the sexual act in order to procreate but also the quality of the spermatozoa produced. Sperm morphology may be so significantly affected as to reduce the chances of fertilization or increase the incidence of having a low birth weight infant. Doyle (1992) and Dickerson (1995) are just two authors that recognize the danger of alcohol consumption during the pre-pregnancy and pregnancy stage. There is still no firm agreement between parties concerned, that is the medical profession, the prospective parents or the alcohol industries, as to how much alcohol is safe when planning a pregnancy. The consumption of alcohol is socially acceptable in today's society and is linked with the workplace by the fact that several occupations, such as company directors or sales reps, may view wining and dining clients as part of their job and therefore alcohol consumption is not seen as 'drinking', in the context of being a health issue.

There is overriding evidence to support the fact that smoking is one of the major contributors to ill health, not just the cancer-related illnesses but chronic illnesses such as heart, respiratory and circulatory diseases. Women who smoke during pregnancy are at increased risk of delivering a baby which is either preterm or of low birth weight or both. Little attention has been paid until recently to the effects of nicotine upon the sperm, but now evidence exists (Summers & Price 1993) to suggest that the smoking habits of the father should be addressed. Nicotine causes an alteration in spermatogenesis, sperm mobility and sperm morphology. There may also be a link between smoking and chromosomal abnormalities and, although the risk may be minimal, it is still a risk that could be avoided altogether. Rubin et al (1988) and Cnattinguis (1989) also offer supportive evidence that the smoking habits of the prospective father do have a detrimental effect upon the birth weight of the subsequent infant.

A study conducted by Hyssala et al (1992) in Finland on the smoking and drinking habits of future fathers from the onset of their wives' pregnancies concluded that within all categories in relation to level of education, occupation and age there was a reduction in smoking and alcohol consumption during the pregnancy. This had a positive effect upon the outcome of the pregnancy and the future health of the whole family. Healthy lifestyle behaviours in respect of alcohol and smoking were continued after the birth of the baby which had obvious health benefits for the parents and the growing infant.

Social class

It is a well-recognized fact that lifestyle behaviours and social class are intertwined. The social class that people occupy has an effect upon many spheres of their lives and the impact upon health cannot be denied. The lower social classes do not fare well in the health market, which may be because they are not inclined to make use of preventive health services nor are they in a position to utilize the health services to their best advantage. One service which is not often used by prospective parents is preconception care. This service is mainly available in the private sector of the health market and therefore only accessible to the higher social classes who are in a position to pay for it. There are few formalized NHS clinics but preconception care is frequently undertaken by nurses and midwives in GP surgeries or family planning clinics or in partnership with doctors who have an interest in this area of health. The value of preconception care counselling cannot be overstressed, especially if a couple are having difficulty in conceiving or have already had an obstetric tragedy. This area of health education may highlight some simple adjustment to lifestyle behaviour, such as reducing the amount of alcohol consumed, in order to achieve a conception.

Age of prospective parents

Due to an overall improvement in people's lives, we as a nation are living longer and healthier lives. It used to be thought that the optimum age for the woman to conceive was in her early 20s, when she was at her peak health, but that is not necessarily the case today. Many women are delaying pregnancy until they are in their mid 30s which, because of improved health and lifestyle, does not generally present any increase in maternal and perinatal morbidity or mortality. The age of the mother at conception has alway caused concern in relation to abnormalities in the offspring, particularly Down's syndrome, and it was always assumed that the age of the father was not significant and that he was capable of fathering a healthy infant at an advanced age. However, there is some evidence to suggest that advanced paternal age may be linked with new single gene mutations in the offspring (Vogel 1983). Achondroplasia, Marfan's syndrome and neurofibromatosis are just three examples. This is worthy of consideration and perhaps investigation in view of the serious consequences.

At the other end of the spectrum, we have the adolescent father. Adolescence itself is often a time of great emotional and psychological change, coupled with the physical developments that are also taking place. Adolescence is a time of transition between childhood and adulthood and is not the best time to embark upon the difficult journey to becoming a father. The majority of teenage pregnancies are unplanned and therefore unprepared for to the extent that is necessary. It is perhaps for this reason that the adolescent father is often viewed as being uncaring, uninterested and lacking in paternal responsibility (Taucher 1991), although earlier work done by Vaz et al (1983) disputes this. From a sociological perspective adolescent fatherhood may be seen, in a perverse kind of way, as being an achievement. Often adolescent fathers are from the lower socioeconomic group who fail to achieve well at school and have limited choice in the employment market and therefore have low expectations of achievement and low self-esteem. The status that fatherhood brings with it heightens their self-esteem and gives them a sense of accomplishment. Several authors (Lorenzi et al 1977, Caparulo & London 1981, Barret & Robinson 1986, Rivara et al 1986, Robinson 1988) report that the majority of adolescent fathers are proud and excited about becoming a father, that financial support for the baby is maintained and contact with their girlfriend and the baby is maintained for at least the first year of the baby's life. This, of course, is a very short time when one considers the number of years that a parent is responsible for a child. However, it is acknowledged that adolescent fathers may have greater difficulty in adapting to their new role of being a parent and accepting the responsibility that goes with it than older fathers.

THE TRANSITION TO FATHERHOOD

The transition to fatherhood can be a traumatic experience for some and unfortunately there is little preparation for it. Attention has focused predominantly on the woman and the emotional and psychological adjustments that she will inevitably make, with little thought being given to the adaptations that the man will have to make. Women experience the physical changes and adaptations that pregnancy brings in order to prepare them for the impending birth of their baby. Men do not have any physical preparation, unless they experience couvade symptoms, which are restricted to the minority of fathers. It has been suggested by Watson et al (1995) that men and women become parents at the same time but not necessarily in the same way. Men do not experience the physical changes that their female partners undergo but the majority of men do acknowledge a change in their sense of responsibility and how they view themselves. This can sometimes be an isolating experience which may lead to depression in the father in the postnatal period, as documented by Ballard & Davies (1996).

A proportion of men, often the higher social classes, do participate actively in the childbirth experience by attending antenatal and parentcraft classes and also by being with their partner during the labour process in order to offer support. However, although men are often a good support to their partners during labour and on the whole find the event wonderful, some may experience feelings of uselessness. Men who attend parentcraft classes with their partner are more prepared as to what their role during labour entails and how best to support their partner through this experience in order to make it emotionally and psychologically satisfying for them both.

It is perhaps the more intimate and personal nature of becoming a father that causes most trauma. The issues that men often leave unsaid can cause great concern, such as ensuring financial stability, embracing the enormous responsibility that fatherhood brings with it or sometimes the change in sexual relationship with their partner. It is becoming increasingly recognized that fathers experience many emotions during this transitionary phase of their lives and require skilled help and understanding (Chalmers & Meyer 1996). These emotions often parallel the childbirth process, that is, antenatal, intrapartum and postpartum phases.

Often, the antenatal phase is viewed as a decision-making time by the man. If the woman was in full-time paid employment and decides to leave work altogether to care for the infant, this will have obvious financial implications not just for the daily running of the household but particularly for the social and leisure side of life. The increasing financial demands that the new baby will undoubtedly bring to the family mean that nights out and holidays may have to be foregone until financial stability has returned. It is often accepted as part of having a baby in this day and age that the extras will have to be given up so that the couple can become parents but some men may actually resent having to give up the prospect of a new car or a holiday in favour of a baby.

During the labour phase of the childbirth process, men are seen as the providers of support for their partners and are encouraged to participate. It must, however, be recognized that although most fathers want to support their partners through this often arduous experience some do not wish to be present at the actual delivery of the infant. A father who is persuaded against his better judgement to be at the delivery may suffer the consequences of what may be viewed in the puerperium as a traumatic experience.

The postnatal period is a time to foster the parent–infant relationship but, sadly, it may also bring great sadness and emotional instability. The man may feel left out because of the demands that the baby places on the mother, in terms of physical and emotional needs. This adjustment period can be very difficult for some parents and may manifest itself in marital disharmony and mental ill health. Postnatal depression in women is recognized as a consequence of childbirth although a great many sufferers go undetected and therefore unhelped. There is now evidence (Ballard & Davies 1996) that fathers may also experience similar mental ill health due to changing roles and responsibilities. It is only in the past 10 years, according to Verkaik (1995), that the medical profession has recognized that men may be susceptible to postnatal depression. Men may experience similar delusions, paranoia and suicidal thoughts as women who suffer from postnatal depression. A great many go undetected by the professionals due to the newness of this illness and men's reluctance to admit to depressive thoughts and feelings at a time when great joy and fulfilment are the expected sentiments.

So how can health professionals ease the transition into fatherhood in order to foster a healthy and happy family unit? The role of the midwife is clearly defined in so much as midwives are the prime caregivers to women and their partners undergoing a normal childbirth process. However, what is not so clearcut is whose responsibility is it to educate men about such matters as parenting.

Attitudes and traditions are absorbed at a very early age. Socialization begins as soon as the baby is born, in that female infants are dressed in pinks and male infants in blue. This socialization continues through the early learning years at school, with girls and boys playing with gender-specific toys and behaving as their gender dictates. Nowadays the boundaries are becoming less defined and girls and boys are beginning to cross into each other's social areas but boys are still expected not to show their feelings whereas girls are expected to be more sensitive and nurturing. More of a conscious effort must be made by all concerned with the early development and socialization of children to change this stereotypical view.

The school curriculum has aspects of sex education and personal and social health included within it, although to what degree is dependent upon the school and the school governors. This is the point at which to start planting the seeds of healthy parenting, for both sexes. It can no longer be seen as the sole responsibility of the female; it has to be seen as a shared responsibility and commitment. It is only through educating young adults in matters of health, relationships, contraception and safe sexual practices that the male's role in becoming a healthy responsible parent will develop. The debate about who should undertake this educational task will no doubt continue but although various health professionals claim that it is their domain, it really requires a team approach from all health professionals involved, such as midwives, school nurses and health visitors.

Midwives become involved when the conception has been confirmed and the pregnancy is a reality. The focus of attention is understandably the mother as she is the vessel which will nurture the developing embryo. The father also needs attention because although he cannot feel the physical changes and adaptations that his partner's body is undergoing, he nevertheless has other adaptations and concerns that need addressing. He may be unsure about his relationship with his partner and how this will change when parenthood is achieved and he will no doubt be anxious, if not scared, about the degree of responsibility that becoming a father will place upon him.

The midwife is in the unique position of being able to help the man come to terms with his changing life. Encouraging the man to accompany his partner to antenatal and parentcraft classes will open the way for him to become more actively involved in the childbirth process that he has embarked upon. Adopting this approach will make his becoming involved more acceptable. There is an increasing demand for parentcraft and antenatal classes which are specially designed for special groups of fathers, such as adolescents. Offering such tailor-made classes will enable the health professional to meet individual needs and help the man to adjust to his new role of father.

Labour is the time when the man can provide support, in terms of the physical needs and the emotional and psychological encouragement that his partner will require. Sadly, the man often feels powerless to help his partner through this ordeal. Here again, the skills of the midwife in involving the man in the labour will make him feel a useful part of the team. He needs to be encouraged to perform the physical aspects of caring for his partner, such as rubbing her back or wiping her face, as well as offering emotional and psychological support as required. Should he not wish to be present at the actual delivery, then he should not be forced into it because it may have long-term psychological effects which often manifest as physical inadequacies. He should, however, be invited back into the delivery room when the infant has just been born and his partner is holding the baby. This will have a more positive and cementing effect upon the newly created family unit in terms of relationship formation. A bad labour experience for the man often spills over into the postnatal period, creating psychological as well as physical maladaptations. The postnatal period is a time when new emotional and physical skills have to be acquired quickly and having to cope with traumatic events which may have occurred during labour does not start the new father off in the best frame of mind.

Nowadays, baby care skills are generally not learnt within the family unit because of the growth of the nuclear family and the reduction in family size, so therefore it falls to the midwives to educate the young parents in child care skills. This process continues with the involvement of the health visitor. The midwife has a responsibility to care for the newly delivered mother and her baby, which obviously includes the father, for a period of not more than 28 days postdelivery, after which time the midwife hands over care of the family to the health visitor. In order to provide good primary care in a holistic manner to the new family unit, it is essential that there is communication between these two health professionals.

Helping the man to become a healthy father cannot be undertaken by one body of health professionals; it has to be a multifaceted approach. Beginning after conception is too late as the optimum health for fatherhood will not be achieved. Education, understanding and recognition of the effect that being a parent has upon the man and the extent of his role and responsibilities will help to promote fatherhood in a positive light. Involving the father in every aspect of the childbirth process and including him in any decision making will foster a feeling of control and partnership. Perhaps there is a need for a support group for fathers so that experiences and fears can be discussed with like-minded people. Lay people's support groups can offer the best kind of help from people who understand and can sympathize.

Perhaps the way forward is to start the change socialization process at birth and to continue through the early years to develop the more caring and sensitive side of young men and make it more acceptable to show their emotions without fear of retribution. It is only through education and choice that the male will grow and develop into an active, participatory and healthy father to his children and the husband that the mother needs.

CONCLUSION

The role of a father is often embarked upon with very little thought or preparation. The majority of pregnancies are unplanned and therefore are unprepared for. Western culture dictates that heterosexual couples will procreate and become parents, but this often overwhelming responsibility is not afforded the time or commitment that it deserves. The level and type of support required by both the new parents varies, due to a couple's individual needs and circumstances but also in relation to whether this is the first baby or a subsequent baby.

As a nation we are generally fitter and healthier which is obviously of great benefit in general health terms, but also in planning a pregnancy. Many of the lifestyle issues that may affect the outcome of a healthy baby can be addressed to minimize the risk. The increased level of education on health and lifestyle means that people are generally more knowledgeable and aware of risks and are therefore more able to avoid or minimize their exposure to them. Schools are the place to begin educating future fathers in aspects of health and to include the wider arena of relationship formation and responsibility. Educating the young on safe sexual practices will help to achieve the Health of the Nations target set to reduce the number of teenage pregnancies by the year 2000 (DoH 1993).

First-time fathers often feel jealous and excluded from their infants because the mother provides most of the infant's needs. However, if they are encouraged to participate actively in their new role by undertaking some of the child care activities then these feelings often subside, making fatherhood a more rewarding experience (Henderson & Brouse 1991). It appears that the level of involvement in the practical aspects of caring for a new baby is again dependent upon whether this is the first baby or not. Evidence suggests (Rustia & Abbott 1993) that first-time fathers are more involved than multiple-time fathers. One of the reasons for this is that parents are more experienced on subsequent births and therefore the necessary level of support in terms of physical skills and psychological adaptation is less.

There is also recognition of the value of fatherhood and the role that fathers play in their child's psychological, emotional and cognitive development (Dragonas et al 1992).

Parents only learn to become parents by trial and error as babies do not come with a manual but, rewardingly, they are all little individuals in their own unique way.

REFERENCES

Ballard C, Davies R 1996 Postnatal depression in fathers. International Review of Psychiatry 8: 65–71

Barret R, Robinson B 1986 Adolescent fathers: often forgotten parents. Paediatric Nursing 12 (4): 273–277

Bozett F W, Hanson S M H 1991 Fatherhood and families in cultural context. Focus on men, vol 6. Springer, New York

Bushy A, Graner R 1990 Innovations in family and community health. Family Community Health 13(3): 82–84

Caparulo F, London K 1981 Adolescent fathers: adolescents first, fathers second. Issues in Health Care of Women 3: 23–33

Chalmers B, Meyer D 1996 What men say about pregnancy, birth and parenthood. Journal of Psychosomatic Obstetrics and Gynecology 17: 47–52

Cnattinguis S 1989 Smoking habits in early pregnancy. Addictive Behaviours 14: 453–457

Dickerson J 1995 Good preconception care starts in school. Modern Midwife November: 15–18

DoH 1993 The health of the nation. The contribution of nurses, midwives and health visitors. Department of Health, London

Doyle W 1992 Preconceptional care – who needs it? Modern Midwife January/February: 18–22

Dragonas T, Thorpe K, Golding J 1992 Transition to fatherhood: a cross cultural comparison. Journal of Psychosomatic Obstetrics and Gynecology 13: 1–19

Henderson A K, Brouse A J 1991 The experiences of new fathers during the first 3 weeks of life. Journal of Advanced Nursing 16: 293–298

Hyssala L, Rautava P, Sillanpaa M, Tuominen J 1992 Changes in the smoking and drinking habits of future fathers from the onset of their wives' pregnancy. Journal of Advanced Nursing 17: 849–854

Kuller J A 1994 Preconceptional counseling and intervention. Archives of Internal Medicine 154: 2273–2280

Lorenzi E, Klerman L, Jekel J 1977 School-age parents: how permanent a relationship? Adolescence 12 (45): 13–22

Mackay W C 1985 Fathering behaviors. The dynamics of the man–child bond. Plenum Press, New York

Rivara F, Sweeney P, Henderson B 1986 Black teenage fathers: what happens when the child is born? Paediatrics 78: 151–158

Robarts P J 1989 Preconceptual care. British Journal of Family Planning 15: 41–43

Robinson B 1988 Teenage pregnancy from the father's perspective. American Journal of Orthopsychiatry 58 (1): 46–51

Rubin D, Krasilnikopp P, Leventhal J, Berget A, Weile B 1988 Cigarette smoking and alcohol consumption during pregnancy by Danish women and their spouses. A potential source of fetal morbidity. American Journal of Drug and Alcohol Abuse 14: 405–441

Rustia J G, Abbott D 1993 Father involvement in infant care: two longitudinal studies. International Journal of Nursing Studies 30 (6): 467–476

Savitz E D A, Whelan E A, Kleckner R C 1989 Effect of parents' occupational exposures on risk of stillbirth, preterm delivery, and small-for-gestational-age infants. Americal Journal of Epidemiology 129: 1201–1218

Summers L, Price R A 1993 Preconception care. An opportunity to maximize health in pregnancy. Journal of Nurse-Midwifery 38(4)

Taskinen H, Anttila A, Lindbohm M et al 1989 Spontaneous abortions and congenital malformations among the wives of men occupationally exposed to organic solvents. Scandinavian Journal of Work Environment and Health 15: 345–352

Taucher P 1991 Support for the adolescent father. Nursing Forum 26 (1): 22–26

Vaz R, Smolen P, Miller C 1983 Adolescent pregnancy: involvement of the male partner. Journal of Adolescent Health Care 4 (4): 246–250

Verkaik R 1995 Men with the baby blues. Style December 31: 18–19

Vogel F 1983 Mutation in man. In: Emory A E, Rimoin E L (eds) Principles and practice of medical genetics. Churchill Livingstone, New York

Watson W, Watson L, Wetzel W, Bader E, Talbot Y 1995 Transition to parenthood: what about fathers? Canadian Family Physician 41: 807–811

Webb C 1994 Living sexuality. Issues for nursing and health. Scutari Press/Royal College of Nursing, London

7

Men and heart disease

Judith Ormrod

INTRODUCTION

A major cause of mortality in much of the industrialized world is ischaemic heart disease. In 1996 ischaemic heart disease ranked first with 7.2 million deaths worldwide whilst cerebrovascular disease was ranked second with 4.6 million deaths worldwide (WHO 1997). However, over twice as many deaths occurred due to cerebrovascular disease in developing countries as in the industrialized countries (WHO 1997).

Within this chapter the major causes of ischaemic heart disease will be considered together with emerging or potential risk factors as well as the major forms of treatment. It may be no surprise that a great deal of research into the risk factors of ischaemic heart disease has been carried out primarily due to the mortality and morbidity incurred worldwide. However, the majority of research studies cited tend to be from Western Europe and North America. During the 1960s and 1970s the subject population tended to be white middle-class males but latterly other groups, such as women and people of colour, have also been considered.

The major risk factors which will be discussed are smoking, hypertension, physical activity and obesity, psychosocial risk factors, diabetes mellitus and hypercholesterolaemia.

SMOKING

Lung cancer is the disease most commonly associated with cigarette smoking. In 1995, lung cancer deaths attributed to cigarette smoking amounted to 514 000 whilst 625 000 deaths from heart and vascular disease were attributed to smoking in the same year in the United Kingdom (WHO 1997).

In industrialized countries it is estimated that 42% of men and 24% of women smoke, whilst it appears that individuals are commencing smoking at a younger age (median 15) in developed countries (WHO 1997). This tends to reduce the age at which death from smoking-related illnesses occurs but also increases the risk (Doll et al 1994). If individuals commence their smoking at an early age it may prove extremely difficult to stop. For those who continue to smoke throughout their lives, it has been estimated that 50% will die from smoking-related causes. Half of these deaths will occur between the ages of 35 and 69 and the second half at 70 years and upwards (Peto et al 1994).

Smokers have an increased risk of sudden cardiac death, being 2–4 times the risk of non-smokers (Glantz & Parmley 1991). The risk increases with the number of cigarettes smoked, heavy smokers (the author has been unable to find an appropriate definition) apparently having 2–3 times the death rate of non-smokers (Glantz & Parmley 1991). Individuals who may be termed passive smokers in that they have never smoked but are subject to environmental tobacco smoke are also at risk. A meta-analysis and two prospective trials have calculated the risk of cardiovascular disease as being 1.2–1.3 for those exposed to environmental tobacco smoke (Glantz & Parmley 1991, Steenland et al 1996, Kawachi et al 1997, Howard et al 1998).

However, whilst these figures may appear alarmist the cessation of cigarette smoking can reduce the risks. Estimates of reduced risk vary, mainly in connection with the study under review but also the lack of consistent measuring tools used by the researchers.

The most optimistic in regard to benefits of smoking cessation appears to be the British Doctors Study (Doll & Peto 1976) in which excess risk was considered to have halved within 2–3 years and by 10 years the risk was reduced to that of a non-smoker.

The results from the British Regional Heart Study are not so optimistic (Cook et al 1986) in that they considered the reduction in risk to be more gradual and found that men who had given up smoking at least 10 years ago still had an increased risk in comparison with non-smokers. However, in relation to secondary prevention, the cessation of smoking following a myocardial infarction offers substantial benefits.

In Daly et al's (1983) study, they found that stopping smoking following a myocardial infarction halved the number of cardiovascular deaths and also the number of non-fatal recurrences over a 14-year period.

Rose & Colewell's (1992) 14-year follow-up study of individuals who had suffered a myocardial infarction highlighted a 37% mortality in those who had stopped smoking in comparison with an 82% mortality in those individuals who had continued to smoke.

It therefore appears imperative to continue to inform people on an individual and community level of the dangers. Also, for those who have suffered a myocardial infarction and wish to cease smoking, individual help needs to be made more widely available.

HYPERTENSION

Hypertension appears to be a major contributor to ischaemic heart disease and also increases the risk of reinfarction and coronary mortality following an initial myocardial infarction (Connolly et al 1983, Wong et al 1989).

Following the fifth report of the Joint National Committee on Detection, Evaluation and Treatment of High Blood Pressure in 1993, a new classification has been agreed. Hypertension may be defined as a systolic BP of 140 mmHg or greater and a diastolic BP of 90 mmHg or greater. There are also considered to be three stages: stage 1 – systolic BP (SBP) 140–159 mmHg and diastolic BP (DBP) 90–99 mmHg to stage 3 – SBP >180 mmHg and/or DBP >110 mmHg. Furthermore, hypertension may be classified as complicated or uncomplicated depending on the presence or absence of target organ manifestations which may include peripheral vascular disease, cardiac, retinal, renal or cerebrovascular disease.

Risk is directly associated with the blood pressure level and the presence of target organ involvement. In the case of cardiovascular risk factors, these include left ventricular hypertrophy, glucose intolerance and hypercholesterolaemia.

It is also important to note that during a 12-year follow-up study of approximately 350 000 middle-aged men involved in the Multiple Risk Factor Intervention Trial, 32% of the deaths attributed to ischaemic heart disease related to elevated BP occurred in individuals whose BP was below the level at which pharmacological treatment would have been prescribed (Stamler et al 1993b).

The multiple causes of hypertension include obesity, lack of exercise, elevated sodium intake, increased alcohol intake, low intakes of magnesium, calcium and potassium and chronic stress (Cutler et al 1997). This has led to a large number of research studies being undertaken using non-pharmacological approaches. Weight loss and exercise, especially low intensity/high frequency, appear to be effective (Fagard 1995, Trials of Hypertension Prevention Collaborative Research Group 1997). Reducing dietary sodium intake by 80–100 mmol/day appears to reduce blood pressure by 5/3 mmHg (systolic/diastolic) in hypertensive individuals (Cutler et al 1997). Also, reducing alcohol intake by 85% (an average of three drinks/day reduced to three drinks/week) (Puddey et al 1985). Other studies have found that increasing dietary potassium (Whetton et al 1997) and lowering saturated fats and dairy produce intake as well as increasing fruit and vegetable intake has also had a positive effect (Appel et al 1997).

But the multiple causes of hypertension do need to be stressed. A number of criticisms may also be levelled at the research studies. The majority of randomized clinical trials considering hypertension prevention have had a small number of subjects and have taken place over a relatively short period of time. Those alterations based on client lifestyle modifications require commitment and whilst the research has highlighted short-term benefits, whether these benefits continue in the long term has not been evaluated.

Many individuals who are hypertensive may require continuous pharmacological treatment over many years. A combination of lifestyle modification together with drug treatment may lead to a reduction in the dosage and potentially the number of hypertensive drugs an individual may need to take.

PHYSICAL ACTIVITY AND OBESITY

The value of increased physical activity and its role in primary and, to a larger extent, secondary prevention of ischaemic heart disease has been studied extensively (Berlin & Colditz 1990, Franklin et al 1991).

Many prospective studies on exercise and cardiovascular mortality highlight higher death rates in those who have a sedentary lifestyle (Blair et al 1989, Kohl et al 1992). Fletcher et al (1996) have suggested that the sedentary lifestyle of many individuals may be an important coronary risk factor which requires further research. However, the amount, type and frequency of exercise or total kilocalorie output tends to vary in many studies. The effect may differ between middle-aged men and women and the total amount of intensity will vary depending on the outcome measures.

It appears that low-intensity and moderate-intensity activity are effective in reducing the majority of risk factors. However, high-intensity exercise may prove beneficial to those with high-density lipoprotein levels and those with hypertension (Blair et al 1989, 1991).

Other studies have considered exercise-induced silent myocardial ischaemia in athletes (Katzel et al 1998) and a small-scale study of 25 men with preexisting left ventricular dysfunction and the effect of high-intensity exercise (Dubach et al 1997). They found that high-intensity exercise did not adversely affect the subjects' cardiovascular functioning.

Overall, two important factors need to be considered: any exercise is better than none and a firm commitment is required since the atherosclerotic process is progressive.

Closely associated with physical activity is the concept of maintaining a body weight within the recommended guidelines. The Buffalo Health Study (Dorn et al 1997) investigated the long-term relationship between body mass index and mortality in a random sample of white men and women (611 and 697 respectively) aged 28–96 who were living in the town of Buffalo, New York in 1960. The 29-year follow-up identified increased body mass index as being linked with ischaemic heart disease and cardiovascular disease mortality in younger men and women only.

Another longitudinal study (Suadicani et al 1997) carried out in Copenhagen considered weight changes and the risk of ischaemic heart disease in 2903 men (53–74 years) who were initiated into the study in 1970–71. The results of this 8-year follow-up (following on from the 1985–6 review) found that any alteration in weight from middle age to old age was of little clinical importance to those men who did not already have preexisting cardiovascular disease.

The final study considered is the Whitehall II Study (Stafford et al 1998) which considered 6895 men and 3413 women aged between 35 and 55 who were civil servants in London. The findings highlighted that steady weight change and weight fluctuations had no independent effect on men and ischaemic heart disease. The effects were more apparent in women.

Overall, the three longitudinal studies mentioned, which all involved large sample sizes, appear to confirm that the association between body mass index and cardiovascular mortality is apparent in younger men and women only.

PSYCHOSOCIAL RISK FACTORS

A psychosocial factor may be defined as a psychosocial occurrence which may relate to the social environment and to pathophysiological changes (Hemingway & Marmot 1998). These factors are usually measured by questionnaires. In relation to ischaemic heart disease, there appear to be four general areas which have been extensively investigated. These include depression and anxiety, hostility and type A behaviour, job control and demands, and, lastly, social supports – the buffer theory.

In regard to depression and anxiety the studies undertaken have considered this factor in primary and secondary prevention of ischaemic heart disease. Anxiety and depression are well-defined psychological disorders with a number of reliable and well-validated questionnaires available. The link between anxiety and depression and the incidence of ischaemic heart disease may have a number of methodological hurdles to overcome. The majority of studies since the mid-1980s have been longitudinal and have concentrated on middle-aged men (Hagman et al 1987, Haines et al 1987, Appels and Mulder 1990, Kawachi 1994). The length of time the studies took to complete varies from 2 to 12 years and the ages of the subjects were 40–64 (Kawachi (1994) 42–47 years). The results all highlighted that anxiety and depression were strong predictors of ischaemic heart disease.

The existence of depression and the link with the severity of preexisting ischaemic heart disease was studied by Ahto et al (1997) in Finland. This study consisted of a matched sample of 488 men and 708 women over 64 years. Despite the small sample size the prevalence of depression was 9% higher among the men than the women (29% and 20% respectively). Overall, the researchers felt that depression was common among patients with ischaemic heart disease. They felt that acute or chronic psychic stress related to ischaemic heart disease could potentially explain the incidence of depression. This idea does tend to suggest a few questions. Is pre-existing depression potentially linked with developing heart disease or is depression the consequence of the heart disease, as Ahto et al (1997) suggest?

Hostility and type A behaviour are frequently cited as being major psychosocial risk factors. Males in particular displaying type A behaviour pattern, characterized by impatience, competitive behaviour, rapid speech and a potential for hostility, have been linked with ischaemic heart disease since the early Framingham Study and the Western Collaborative Study (Rosenman et al 1976). Later studies have suggested that the concept of hostility may provide a more direct link than the more nebulous type A behaviour profile. But studies have offered conflicting conclusions. Shekelle et al (1983) followed up 1977 men aged 40–58 years for 20 years and found a strong association between hostility, as measured by the Minnesota Multiphasic Personality Inventory (MMPI), and ischaemic heart disease. Alternatively, Hearn et al (1989) followed up 1399 19-year-old students from Minnesota for 33 years and found no association, as did Barefoot et al (1995), who followed up a mixed sample of men and women aged 50 for 27 years. Marrutan et al (1993) periodically reviewed the health of 620 general medical patients for 20 years and found no association.

Another study by Rancho et al (1997), using a cross-sectional design, matched 279 men aged between 30 and 70 years who had suffered a myocardial infarction with a 'healthy' control group. Whilst the study primarily focused on non-ischaemic heart disease and hostility, it did subdivide the concept of hostility. The three components were resentment, suspicion and aggression. Their results concluded that all components of hostility were related to non-ischaemic heart disease but not to ischaemic heart disease.

The third major area related to psychosocial factors is that of job control. For many years certain occupations were deemed high risk. Latterly interest has been shown in the components of a job which may increase the ischaemic heart disease risk. A 'job strain' model suggests that jobs that allow the individual little control over their work but contain high levels of conflicting demands may lead to high strain.

Three large-scale longitudinal studies have focused on men in steady employment. Johnson et al (1989) studied 19 Swedish men for 9 years.

Alterman et al (1994) studied 1683 men for 25 years and Suadicani et al (1993) studied 1752 men for 3 years. The results tend to vary, with Johnson's (1989) work showing strong positive links whilst Alterman (1994) presented a mixed picture and Suadicani (1993) highlighted that an inability to relax after work was associated with a three-fold increased risk of ischaemic heart disease.

A major British study has been the Whitehall II Study (Stafford et al 1989) which followed 6895 men and 3413 women who were employed by the Civil Service for 5 years. The results were strongly positive in support of the 'job strain' model.

The final psychosocial factor is that of social support. This relates to the number of social contacts an individual has ready access to but also the quality of that support, in that the individual can confide in that person as well as gain emotional support.

Rosengren et al (1996) found in their study of 744 men in Sweden that poor emotional support and social integration could be regarded as independent predictors of mortality from all causes. However, the researchers expressed caution in that the association between these factors and mortality could be due to compounding from other factors.

Watkins et al (1991) explored the concept of male gender role stress and cardiovascular disease amongst employed men. Those scoring high levels experienced undesirable outcomes.

At times it may be difficult for men to obtain social support (Barbee et al 1993, Hobfoll et al 1994). This may be due to gender role expectations in that the male role emphasizes emotional control, autonomy and achievement (Barbee et al 1993). Men may use antisocial actions in social situations (Hobfoll et al 1994).

Lastly, it appears that being married offers some protection for men (Watkins et al 1991). The final two studies considered social support and its effects on men who had already experienced a myocardial infarction. Vogh et al (1992) and Orth-Gomer et al (1993) both found that men who had suffered a myocardial infarction and received support from their spouses experienced more positive outcomes than those who did not have such support. However, in regard to the effect of social support systems, caution needs to be exercised in that there has been little consistency of outcome measures.

DIABETES MELLITUS

Both type 1 and type 2 diabetics are at increased risk for the development of ischaemic heart disease. The increased risk is up to four times greater than non-diabetic subjects (Stamler et al, 1993a). In the Minnesota and Framingham Studies, the risk of reinfarction in diabetes was increased by 50% and the mortality was 40% higher than non-diabetic individuals during long-term follow-up (Wong et al 1989, Sprafka et al 1991). Although in type 1 diabetes it may take 30 years for ischaemic heart disease to manifest itself, the increased risk is generally obvious at the time of presentation with type 2 diabetes (Herman et al 1977). The extent of blood sugar elevation is directly related to cardiovascular risk. In this way, like systemic hypertension and total serum cholesterol, blood sugar level seems to be a continuous risk factor.

The principal mechanisms invoked in order to explain the link between diabetes and cardiovascular disease generally fall into five groups (Gerstein 1998):

1. direct toxic effects of glucose;
2. indirect toxic effects of glucose (i.e. due to inadequate insulin secretion for normoglycaemia);
3. insulin resistance and hyperinsulinaemia;
4. the concurrent development of other IHD risk factors (e.g. hypertension, obesity, hyperlipidaemia);
5. association with other IHD risk factors (e.g. poor socioeconomic status, low birth weight).

Some of the mechanisms are still open to debate (Stern 1995, Jarret 1996).

These data have led to attempts to discover whether modification of blood glucose alters cardiovascular risk. Several trials have suggested that this may be so (Diabetes Control and Complications Trial Research Group 1993, Malmberg et al 1995, Genuth 1996).

The recently published longitudinal study of type 2 diabetes from the UK confirms that a quintet of potentially modifiable risk factors for coronary artery disease exists in these patients. This is one of the largest longitudinal studies, with 3055 white diabetic patients followed up for a mean of 7.9 years; 335 patients developed ischaemic heart disease within 10 years (Turner et al 1998). Other large series, such as the personal series reported by Nabarro (1991), have given an even higher prevalence of coronary heart disease, in up to 19.1% of a series of 4926 patients with type 2 diabetes.

LIPIDS AND ISCHAEMIC HEART DISEASE

A raised serum cholesterol is a major risk factor for IHD (Levine et al 1995, Oliver et al 1995). The level of developing IHD rises absolutely with increasing levels of serum cholesterol (Neaton et al 1992). Before the advent of the 'statin' drugs, the trials of cholesterol lowering were either too small or too weak to demonstrate significant reductions in mortality (Rossouw 1995).

Primary prevention of coronary heart disease by cholesterol reduction strategies presents a potentially huge socioeconomic burden. Expenditure on statin drugs was over £20M in 1993, rising to £113M by 1997 (DoH 1998). Were primary prevention of IHD by aggressive cholesterol level reduction by statins to be implemented, a further huge (and possibly unsustainable) rise in the NHS drug budget would ensue. Population approaches argue that although the risk of developing IHD for any particular individual may be lowered by a small amount, the population effect could be considerable as so many of the population are affected. It has also to be borne in mind that a substantial number of coronary events affect those who are at average risk and would therefore be missed by strategies aimed solely at high-risk individuals. Consequently, UK public health policy is shaped by a mixture of population and high-risk (targeted) individual approaches.

Cholesterol lowering is principally achieved by two types of intervention – diet and drugs. Low-fat diets have received extensive scrutiny but are totally dependent on compliance and how tightly controlled the lipid content of the diet is. In hospital dietary changes can bring substantial reductions in serum cholesterol (Clarke et al 1997) but when applied to the general population at large, only tiny changes are seen; the reduction from lipid-lowering diets is only 1–5% (Neil et al 1995, Brunner et al 1997). The disappointing results of lipid-lowering diets may to some extent be explained by the substitution of complex carbohydrates for fat. This brings down *total* cholesterol, but leaves the LDL:HDL ratio unaffected, thereby failing to reduce the risk of IHD (Clarke et al 1997). In other words, reducing risk of IHD is not just due to lowering of cholesterol levels alone.

Trials of garlic in lowering cholesterol are significantly flawed and the evidence cannot be regarded as useful. The consumption of oats (Rispin et al 1992) or cereals (Olson et al 1997) shows a 2% lowering of cholesterol. Soya protein also causes a small fall in cholesterol levels (Anderson et al 1995).

Drug therapy remains, then, the most effective way of lowering cholesterol levels. Although effective drugs have been around for a long time (e.g. nicotinic acid was shown to reduce cholesterol and triglyceride levels in the 1950s), the introduction of the statins (HMG CoA reductase inhibitors) has completely revolutionized the drug treatment of hypercholesterolaemia.

There are 22 randomized controlled trials of cholesterol lowering and clinical outcomes using these drugs. The overall results show that the statins reduce the risk of death from coronary heart disease by 25%.

Another trial may report soon which may extend the indications for statin therapy. The Air Force/Texas Coronary Atherosclerosis Prevention Study of Lovastatin Trial was stopped prematurely after a 36% reduction in combined fatal and non-fatal IHD endpoints was found (Husten 1990).

The very long-term safety and sustained efficacy of statins has not yet been substantiated. The Standing Medical Advisory Committee (SMAC), a statutory UK committee that advises Ministers, has recently prepared a position statement on the use of statins in patients with known IHD and people at significant risk of developing overt IHD. The appropriate threshold to trigger statin therapy has been suggested as: patients with IHD or people with an abnormal IHD risk of 3% per year or more. This risk is resistant to risk reduction by other means. The SMAC breaks down the priorities for statin treatment into three groups.

1. The first priority for lipid lowering with a statin is patients who have had a myocardial infarction. These patients have a very high IHD risk and treatment is indicated when total cholesterol is as low as 4.8 mmol/l (or LDL as low as 3.2 mmol/l if measured).

2. The second priority for lipid-lowering therapy is patients with angina or other clinically overt atherosclerotic disease who have a total cholesterol of 5.5 mmol/l or more (or LDL of 3.7 mmol/l if measured). This includes patients with peripheral vascular disease or symptomatic carotid disease or who have previously undergone bypass grafting or angioplasty. These patients have a risk of major coronary events of 3% per year.

Together these two priority groups encompass around 4.8% of the population aged 35–69 (5.9% of men and 3.6% of women).

3. The third priority is primary prevention, i.e. the treatment of people without clinical apparent vascular disease but who nevertheless have a high risk of developing overt IHD. Such people may be at risk because of a combination of other IHD risk factors such as familial hyperlipidaemia, diabetes or hypertension. This group encompasses 3.4% of the population aged 35–69 years (5.7% of men and 0.4% of women). Formal estimation of IHD risk is essential when considering primary prevention of IHD. The Sheffield Table is a simple method for identifying those without IHD who should have their cholesterol measured (Ramsey et al 1996).

EMERGING RISK FACTORS

The gradual decline in the incidence of coronary heart disease has been, at least in part, attributed to the control of traditional risk factors for coronary heart disease referred to earlier in this chapter (Jonsilahti et al 1995).

New risk factors are now being described. They include elevated lipoprotein (a) levels, excess iron load, hypercoagulability and homocystenaemia. Angiotensin-converting enzyme inhibitor polymorphism and human white cell leucocyte antigen DR II phenotype status are now also emerging as risk factors (Mehta et al 1998).

Other studies have provided evidence that inflammatory responses may be implicated in the pathogenesis of atherosclerosis (Ross 1993). In addition to inflammation, it is also possible that we may eventually conclude that infection with very common organisms, such as cytomegalovirus (CMV) or chlamydia pneumonia, may lead to localized arterial infection, inflammation and the development of atherosclerosis. This raises the possibility that antibiotics may become part of the treatment strategy for ischaemic heart disease (Gupta et al 1997) and a small UK series has already pointed to a therapeutic role for azithromycin in the treatment of survivors of myocardial infarction (Gupta et al 1997).

Large-scale trials are being planned to critically evaluate this novel strategy.

ETHNICITY

Within the United Kingdom and North America the majority of epidemiological studies into risk factors for IHD have been carried out on white male and frequently middle-class subjects. This appears rather short-sighted.

According to Anand & Yusuf (1998), ethnicity-related research is extremely important for a number of reasons. First, the rates of known risk factors for a disease are documented. New risk factors may be identified, giving clues to differences and similarities in the causes of the disease. Also, the research may lead to specific prevention strategies which are tailored to the major ethnic groups.

An ethnic group refers to a group of people who share common cultural characteristics such as diet, religion and language. Since the differences in rates of disease between populations may be explained by biological, socioeconomic, cultural and genetic factors, it may be more appropriate to consider clarification by ethnic origin rather than race (Anand & Yusuf 1998).

The ethnic variations in rates of disease are closely linked with geographical patterns. The Seven Countries Study (Menotti et al 1997) was one of the first epidemiological studies in which 16 cohorts of men aged 49–59 years were studied over 25 years. Differences in mortality were apparent in that the IHD rates were low in the Mediterranean countries and Japan but were high in the USA and Finland. These differences could be explained by blood pressure, serum cholesterol and diet.

The MONICA Study (MONItoring of trends and determinants in CArdiovascular disease) is a cardiovascular surveillance project taking place in 26 countries. The findings indicate a greater than 14-fold difference between countries in IHD mortality in men and for women more than 11-fold (Siegfried 1989).

The majority of ethnicity-related research has occurred in the USA. The IHD mortality rate in African-American men is 2.4% higher than in white men (American Heart Association 1995). Sudden cardiac deaths are also more common among African-American men (Gillum 1989). The common risk factors of IHD often occur earlier or are more severe in African-American men (American Heart Association 1995). Other American studies have considered younger individuals. The CARDIA Study (Krieger & Sidney 1996) and the PDAY Research Growth Pathological Determinants of Atherosclerosis in Youth (McGill et al 1997) have both found IHD risk factors occurring earlier.

However, as Anand & Yusuf (1998) have stated, the differences in socioeconomic status between African-Americans and whites may lead to fewer interactions with health care services, fewer investigative tests and treatment.

People who originate from South Asia (India, Bangladesh, Pakistan and Sri Lanka) also suffer high mortality (Ersas et al 1992). One British study (Bhatnagar et al 1995) compared the measurable risk factors of individuals living in urban areas in Britain and their siblings living in India. Systolic BP, total cholesterol, fasting glucose and body mass index were all higher in the UK group.

In conclusion, whilst the majority of studies are American and show higher incidence, earlier onset and higher mortality rates of IHD, there appears to be a need to increase the number of studies based on ethnic groups in order primarily to initiate specific prevention strategies.

TREATMENT OPTIONS

Medical treatment, PTCA or CABG for stable coronary heart disease?

The treatment of coronary heart disease can be broadly broken into three options: medical treatment (drugs), percutaneous intervention (PTCA) or coronary artery bypass grafting (CABG). Four major trials provide the basis for current practice (European Coronary Surgery Study Group 1982, Alderman et al 1990, VA Coronary Artery Bypass Surgery Co-operative Study Group 1992, Yusuf et al 1994); although widely quoted and followed, they are in the era of PTCA, stenting, and the widespread use of out of date multiple arterial conduits for coronary revascularization. Comparison of the three major strategies is further compounded by continuous technological evolution in the mechanical strategies and the widespread introduction of new antiplatelet agents and lipid-lowering agents into practice.

PTCA was developed 10 years after CABG had become the alternative to drug therapy for patients with significant ischaemic heart disease. It is important to recognize that PTCA has not replaced CABG and at present is unlikely to do so. PTCA has to a significant extent been used to relieve symptoms in patients with single-vessel disease, whereas the converse is true for CABG – almost all patients have severe multivessel coronary disease.

In the recently published RITA-2 Trial (RITA-2 Participants 1997), it appeared that in patients with low-risk coronary heart disease, PTCA can improve short-term outlook but does not preclude the need for further PTCA or CABG.

Nine major trials (e.g. see the BARI Trial; BARI Investigators 1996) and metaanalysis of 5200 patients with multivessel coronary artery disease or CABG seem to show no clear superiority of one over the other. The low numbers of patients enrolled into those trials fail to show any significant effect on mortality between the two treatment modalities. So, until trials incorporating all three major therapeutic approaches to patients with coronary artery disease are performed, we will not know the answer to the question of which is the best approach (Mark et al 1994). Such trials, if performed, would also have to allow for new interventional techniques such as stenting and for the less invasive surgical procedures now being widely developed.

Thrombolysis

The early discovery that acute coronary occlusion was responsible for most cases of acute myocardial infarction lead to attempts over the last 50 years to translate this pathological finding into effective interventions. The last decade has seen many randomized clinical trials of thrombolysis and these have led to the publication of guidelines for the thrombolytic management of acute myocardial infarction (Task Force of the European Society of Cardiology 1996).

The therapeutic agent used for thrombolytic therapy has varied across Europe and the US. In Europe, streptokinase is predominantly used as first-line therapy, whereas in the US recombinant tissue plasminogen activator (rtPA) is more frequently used. Streptokinase is considerably cheaper than regimes that employ rtPA. How to deliver the thrombolytic in the most optimal way has spawned a number of regimens, most of which are under prospective evaluation (Fuster 1993, Simmons & Arnold 1993, Martin & Kennedy 1994).

Aspirin is central to all regimens but heparin, which is commonly administered, has a weaker evidence base to support its use (ISIS-3 Collaborative Group 1992, Collins et al 1996).

Newer agents which affect platelet function, like aspirin, are now being evaluated. These extremely potent agents show great promise and have already proved their worth in unstable angina, particularly when used in conjunction with PTCA and stenting in the EPIC Trial (1994).

Evidence suggests that these agents (of which around 25 compounds are in various phases of evaluation) may offer the promise of a substantial improvement in the management and outcome of acute ischaemic syndromes.

However, despite effective thrombolytic therapies, it seems that only about one-third of patients with acute myocardial infarction receive thrombolysis, which is often withheld on the grounds of advancing age (Ketley & Woods 1995).

Coronary angioplasty (PTCA) has been successful in opening acutely occluded arteries, both with and without thrombolytic therapy. However, many studies in this area suffer from comparisons with each other, as many different (and therefore non-comparable) regimens are used. The evidence that primary angioplasty for acute myocardial infarction is better than thrombolysis can be found (Michels & Yusuf 1995).

It is also possible to conclude that PTCA is worse than thrombolysis (Tiefenbrunn et al 1995) or that the results of PTCA are no different from standard thrombolytic therapy (GUSTO IIb 1997).

For optimal outcomes using PTCA in acute myocardial infarction, a dedicated primary PTCA programme is required in centres with experience so that good outcomes resulting from large volumes can be achieved. The average delay in thrombolysis (in the USA) is approximately 40 min, whereas inevitably delays in receiving primary PTCA are larger (>2 h). So it may be better to administer thrombolysis as first-line therapy until primary angioplasty becomes a practical proposition for the management of acute myocardial infarction.

CONCLUSION

This chapter has attempted to discuss actual and potential risk factors of ischaemic heart disease incorporating relevant research studies. The studies have been based, for the most part, in Western Europe and the USA using white, male and frequently middle-class subjects. Latterly, researchers have begun to address the needs of younger males, those less socially advantaged, people of colour and women.

The treatment options following the onset of ischaemic heart disease have also been described. Relevant studies have been considered but methodological issues have made comparison of treatment options difficult.

REFERENCES

Ahto M, Isoaho R, Puolijoki H et al 1997 Coronary heart disease and depression in the elderly – a population based study. Family Practice 10(41): 436–445

Alderman E L, Bourassa M G, Cohen L S et al 1990 Ten-year follow up of survival and myocardial infarction in the randomised Coronary Artery Surgery Study. Circulation 82: 1629–1646

Alterman T, Shekelle R B, Vernon S W et al 1994 Decision latitude, psychological demand, job strain and coronary heart disease in the Western Electric Study. American Journal of Epidemiology 139: 620–627

American Heart Association 1995 Heart and stroke facts: 1996 statistical supplement. American Heart Association, Dallas, TX

Anand S S, Yusuf S 1998 Ethnicity and cardiovascular disease. In: Yusuf S, Cairns J A, Camm A J et al (eds) Evidence based cardiology. BMJ Books, London p. 329

Anderson J, Johnstone B, Cook-Newell M 1995 Meta-analysis of the effects of soya protein intake on serum lipids. New England Journal of Medicine 333: 276–282

Appel L J, Moore J, Obarjanek E et al 1997 for the DASH Collaborative Research Group. A clinical trial of the effects of dietary patterns on blood pressure. New England Journal of Medicine 336: 1117–1124

Appels A, Mulder P 1990 Excess fatigue as a precursor of myocardial infarction. European Heart Journal 9: 758–764

Barefoot C J, Harsen S, von der Lieth L et al 1995 Hostility, incidence of acute myocardial infarction and mortality in a sample of older Danish men and women. American Journal of Epidemiology 142: 477–484

Barbee A P, Cunningham M R, Winstead B A et al 1993 Effects of gender role expectations on the social support process. Journal of Social Issues 49(3): 175–190

Berlin J A, Colditz C A 1990 A meta-analysis of physical activity in the prevention of coronary heart disease. American Journal of Epidemiology 132: 612–628

Bhatnagar D, Anand I S, Durrington P N et al 1995 Coronary risk factors in people from the Indian sub-continent living in West London and their siblings in India. Lancet 345: 405–409

Blair S N, Kohl H W III, Paffenbarger R S et al 1989 Physical fitness and all-cause mortality: a prospective study of healthy men and women. Journal of the American Medical Association 62: 2395–2401

Blair S N, Kohl H W III, Barlow L E et al 1991 Physical fitness and all-cause mortality in hypertensive men. Annals of Medicine 23: 307–312

Brunner T, White I, Thorogood M et al 1997 Can dietary interventions change diet in cardiovascular risk factors? A meta-analysis of randomised controlled trials. American Journal of Public Health 87: 1415–1422

Bypass Angioplasty Revascularisation Investigation (BARI) Investigators 1996 Comparison of coronary artery bypass surgery with angioplasty in patients with multivessel disease. New England Journal of Medicine 335: 217–225

Clarke R, Frost C, Collins R et al 1997 Dietary lipids and blood cholesterol: quantitative meta-analysis of metabolic ward studies. British Medical Journal 314: 112–117

Collins R, MacMahon S, Flather M et al 1996 Clinical effects of anticoagulant therapy in suspected acute myocardial infarction; a systematic overview of randomised trials. British Medical Journal 313: 652–659

Connolly D C, Elveback L K, Oxman H A 1983 Coronary heart disease in residents of Rochester, Minnesota 1950–1975. III Effect of Hypertension and its treatment on survival of patients with coronary artery disease. Mayo Clinic Proceedings 58(4): 249–254

Cook D G, Pocock S J, Shaper A G et al 1986 Giving up smoking and the risk of heart attacks. Lancet 2: 1376–1380

Cutler J A, Follmann D, Allender P S 1997 Randomised trials of sodium reduction: an overview. American Journal of Nutrition 65: 643S–651S

Daly L T, Mulcahy R, Graham I M, Hickey M 1983 Long term effect on mortality of stopping smoking after unstable angina and myocardial infarction. British Medical Journal 287: 324–326

DoH 1998 Statistics division. Prescription cost analysis system. Effective Health Care 4(3): 3

Diabetes Control and Complications Trial Research Group 1993 The effect of intensive treatment of diabetes on the development and progress of long term complications in insulin-dependent diabetes mellitus. New England Journal of Medicine 329: 977–986

Doll R, Peto R 1976 Mortality in relation to smoking: 20 years observation of British male doctors. British Medical Journal 4: 1525–1536

Doll R, Peto R, Wheatley K et al 1994 Mortality in relation to smoking: 40 years observation of male British doctors. British Medical Journal 309: 901–911

Dorn J M, Schisterman E F, Winkelsten W et al 1997 Body mass index and mortality in a general population sample of men and women: the Buffalo Health Study. American Journal of Epidemiology 145(11): 919–931

Dubach P, Myers J, Dziickan G et al 1997 Effects of high intensity exercise training on central hemodynamic responses to exercise in men with reduced left ventricular function. Journal of the American College of Cardiology 29(7): 1591–1598

EPIC Investigators 1994 Use of monoclonal antibody directed against platelet glycoprotein IIb/IIa receptor in high risk angioplasty. New England Journal of Medicine 330: 956–961

Ersas E A, Yusuf S, Mehta J 1992 Prevalence of coronary heart disease in Asian Indians. American Journal of Cardiology 70: 945–949

European Coronary Surgery Study Group 1982 Long term results of prospective randomised study of coronary artery bypass surgery in stable angina pectoris. Lancet ii: 1173–1180

Fagard R 1995 Prescription and results of physical activity. Journal of Cardiovascular Pharmacology 25 (suppl 1): S20–S27

Fletcher G F, Balady G, Froelicher U F et al 1996 Exercise standards. A statement for healthcare professionals from the American Heart Association. Circulation 86: 340–344

Franklin B A, Bonzheim K, Gordon S et al 1991 Resistance training in cardiac rehabilitation. Journal of Cardiopulmonary Rehabilitation II: 99–106

Fuster V 1993 Coronary thrombolysis: a perspective for the practising physician. New England Journal of Medicine 329: 723–725

Genuth S 1996 Exogenous insulin administration and cardiovascular risk in NIDDM and IDDM. Annals of Internal Medicine 124: 104–109

Gerstein H C 1998 Glucose abnormalities and cardiovascular disease: 'dysglycaemia' as an emerging cardiovascular risk factor. In: Yusuf S, Cairns J, Camm A J et al (eds) Evidence based cardiology. BMJ Books, London pp. 239–250

Gillum R F 1989 Sudden coronary death in the United States 1980–1985. Circulation 79: 756–765

Glantz S A, Parmley W W 1991 Passive smoking and heart disease: epidemiology, physiology and biochemistry. Circulation 83: 1–2

Global Use of Strategies to Open Occluded Coronary Arteries in Acute Coronary Syndromes (Gusto IIb) Angioplasty Substudy Investigators 1997 A clinical trial comparing primary coronary angioplasty with tissue plasminogen activator for acute myocardial infarction. New England Journal of Medicine 336: 1621–1628

Gupta S, Leatham E W, Carrington D et al 1997 Elevated Chlamydia pneumonia antibodies, cardiovascular events and azithromycin in male survivors of acute myocardial infarction. Circulation 96: 404–407

Hagman M, Wilhelmsen L, Wedel H et al 1987 Risk factors for angina pectoris in population study of Swedish men. Journal of Chronic Disability 40: 265–275

Haines A P, Imesm J D, Meade T W 1987 Phobic anxiety and ischaemic heart disease. British Medical Journal 295: 297–299

Hearn M, Murray D M, Luepker R B 1989 Hostility, coronary heart disease and total mortality: a 38 year follow up study of university students. Journal of Behavioural Medicine 12: 105–121

Hemingway H, Marmot M 1998 Psycho-social factors in the primary and secondary prevention of coronary heart disease: a systematic review. In: Yusuf S, Cairns J A, Camm A J et al (eds) Evidence based cardiology. BMJ Books, London, p. 270

Herman J B, Medalic J H, Goldbout U 1977 Differences in cardiovascular morbidity and mortality between previously known and newly diagnosed adults diabetes. Diabetologia 13: 229–234

Hobfoll S F, Dunahoo C L, Ben-Porant Y et al 1994 Gender and coping: the dual axis model of coping. American Journal of Community Psychology 22(1): 49–82

Howard G, Wagenknecht L F, Buxke G L et al 1998 Cigarette smoking and progression of atherosclerosis: the Atherosclerosis Risk in Communities (ARIC) Study. Journal of the American Medical Association 279: 119–124

Husten L 1990 Latest trial on statins shows large benefits for wide range of patients. Lancet 350: 1525

ISIS-3 Collaborative Group 1992 A randomised comparison of streptokinase vs tissue plasminogen activator vs antistreptase and of aspirin vs aspirin alone among 41,299 cases of suspected acute myocardial infarction. Lancet 339: 753–770

Jarrett R J 1996 The cardiovascular risk associated with impaired glucose tolerance. Diabetic Medicine 13(3 supplement 2) 515–519

Johnson J U, Hall E M, Theorell T 1989 Combined effects of job strain and social isolation on cardiovascular disease morbidity and mortality in a random sample of Swedish male working population. Scandinavian Journal of Work and Environmental Health 15: 27–29

Jonsilahti P, Vartainen E, Thornlehto J et al 1995 Effect of risk factors and changes in risk factors on coronary mortality in three cohorts of middle-aged people in eastern Finland. American Journal of Epidemiology 141: 50–60

Kawachi I, Sparrow D, Vokonas P S, Welss S T 1994 Symptoms of anxiety and coronary heart disease. Circulation 90: 2225–2229

Katzel L I, Fleg J L, Burby-Whithead M J et al 1998 Exercise induced silent myocardial ischaemia in master athletes. American Journal of Cardiology 81(3): 261–265

Kawachi I, Colditz G A, Speezer F E et al 1997 A prospective study of passive smoking and coronary heart disease. Circulation 95: 2374–2379

Ketley D, Woods K L 1995 Age limits the use of thrombolytic drugs for acute myocardial infarction in most European countries. European Heart Journal 16 (abstr. suppl): 10

Kohl H W, Gordon N F, Villegan J A et al 1992 Cardio-respiratory fitness, glycaemic status and mortality risk in men. Diabetes Care 15: 184–192

Krieger N, Sidney S 1996 Racial discrimination and blood pressure: the CARDIA Study of young black and white adults. American Journal of Public Health 86(10): 1370–1378

Levine G N, Keaney J F, Vita J A 1995 Cholesterol reduction in cardiovascular disease: clinical benefits and possible mechanisms. New England Journal of Medicine 332(8): 512–521

Malmberg K, Tyden L, Efendic S et al 1995 Randomised trial of insulin-glucose infusion followed by subcutaneous treatment in diabetic patients with acute myocardial infarctions (DIGAMI Study): effects of mortality at 1 year. Journal of the American Colleges of Cardiology 26: 57–65

Mark D B, Nelson C L, Califf R M et al 1994 Continuing evolution of therapy for coronary artery disease. Initial results from the era of coronary angioplasty. Circulation 89: 2015–2025

Marrutan T, Hamburgen M T, Jennings C A et al 1993 Keeping hostility in perspective: coronary heart disease and the hostility scale on the Minnesota Multiphasic Personality Inventory. Mayo Clinic Proceedings SO 68: 109–114

Martin G U, Kennedy J W 1994 Choice of thrombolytic agent. In: Julian D, Braunwald E (eds) Management for acute myocardial infarction. W B Saunders, London pp. 71–105

McGill H R J, McMahon C A, Malcolm G T et al 1997 Effects of serum lipoproteins and smoking on atherosclerosis in young men and women. The PDAY Research Group Pathological Determinants of Atherosclerosis in Youth. Atherosclerosis, Thrombosis and Vascular Biology 17(1): 95–106

Mehta J L, Saleen T G P, Rand I C 1998 Interactive role of infection, inflammation and traditional risk factors in atherosclerosis and coronary artery disease. Journal of the American College of Cardiology 31: 1217–1225

Menotti A, Blackburn H, Kromhout D et al 1997 Changes in population cholesterol levels and coronary heart disease deaths in seven countries. European Heart Journal 18(4): 566–571

Michels K B, Yusuf S 1995 Does PTCA in acute myocardial infarction affect mortality and reinfarction rates? A quantitative overview (meta-analysis) of randomised clinical trials. Circulation 91: 476–485

Nabarro J D N 1991 Diabetes in the United Kingdom: a personal series. Diabetic Medicine 8(1): 59–68

Neaton J D, Blackburn H, Jacobs D et al 1992 Serum cholesterol and mortality: findings for men screened in the Multiple Risk Factor Intervention Trial. Archives of Internal Medicine 152: 1490–1500

Neil H A W, Row L, Godlee R J et al 1995 Randomised controlled trial of lipid lowering advice in general practice. The effects on serum lipids, lipoproteins and antioxidants. British Medical Journal 310: 569–573

Olson B H, Anderson S M, Becker M P et al 1997 Psyllium-enriched cereals lower blood total cholesterol and LDL cholesterol, but not the HDL cholesterol in hypercholesterolaemic adults: results of a meta-analysis. Journal of Nutrition 127: 1973–1980

Orth-Gomer K, Rosengren A, Wilhelmsen L 1993 Lack of social support and incidence of coronary heart disease in middle-aged Swedish men. Psychosomatic Medicine 55: 37–43

Peto R, Lopez A D, Boreham J et al 1994 Mortality from smoking in developed countries 1950–2000. Oxford University Press, Oxford

Puddey I B, Berlin L J, Vandongen K et al 1985 Evidence for a direct effect of alcohol consumption on blood pressure in normotensive men: a randomised controlled trial. Hypertension 7: 707–713

Ramsey L E, Haq I U, Jackson P R et al 1996 The Sheffield Table for primary prevention of coronary heart disease. Lancet 348: 387–388, 1251–1252

Rancho A U, Sanderman R, Bouma J et al 1997 An exploration of the relation between hostility and disease. Journal of Behavioural Medicine 20(3): 223–240

Report of a task force of the European Society of Cardiology 1996 Acute myocardial infarction; pre-hospital and in-hospital management. European Heart Journal 17: 43–63

RITA-2 Participants 1997 Coronary angioplasty versus medical therapy for angina: the second Randomised Intervention Treatment of Angina (RITA-2) Trial. Lancet 350: 461–468

Rispin C, Keenan J, Jacobs O et al 1992 Oat products and lipid lowering: a meta-analysis. Journal of the American Medical Association 267: 3317–3325

Rose G, Colwell L 1992 Randomised controlled trial of anti-smoking advice. Journal of Epidemiology and Community Health 46: 75–77

Rosengren A, Orth-Gomer K, Wedel H et al 1996 Low serum cholesterol, social support and predictors of mortality in middle aged men. A study of men born in 1993. Cardiovascular Risk Factors 6(6): 345–353

Rosenman R H, Brand R J, Sholtz R I et al 1976 Multivariate prediction of coronary heart disease during 8.5 year follow-up in Western Collaborative Group Study. American Journal of Cardiology 37: 903–909

Ross R 1993 The pathogenesis of atherosclerosis: a perspective for the 1990's. Nature 362: 801–809

Rossouw J E 1995 Lipid lowering interventions in angiographic trials (meta-analysis). American Journal of Cardiology 76: 86C–92C

Shekelle R B, Gale M, Ostfeld A M et al 1983 Hostility, risk of coronary heart disease and mortality. Psychosomatic Medicine 45: 109–114

Siegfried B 1989 WHO MONICA Project: objectives and design. International Journal of Epidemiology 18: S29–S37

Simmons M L, Arnold A E 1993 Tailored thrombolytic therapy: a perspective. Circulation 88: 2556–2564

Sprafka J M, Burke G L, Folsom A R, McGoven P G, Hahn L P 1991 Trends in prevalence of diabetes mellitus in patients with myocardial infarction and effects of diabetes on survival. The Minnesota Heart Survey. Diabetes Care 14(7): 537–543.

Stafford M, Hemingway H, Marmot M 1998 Current obesity, steady weight change and weight fluctuations as predictors of physical functioning in middle aged office workers: the Whitehall II Study. International Journal of Obesity and Related Metabolic Disorders 22(1): 23–31

Stamler J, Vaccaro O, Neaton J D et al 1993a Diabetes, other risk factors and 12 year cardio-vascular mortality for men screened in the Multiple Risk Factor Intervention Trial. Diabetes Care 16: 434

Stamler J, Stamler R, Neaton J 1993b Blood pressure, systolic and diastolic and cardiovas-cular risks: US population data. Archives of Internal Medicine 153: 596–615

Steenland K, Thun M, Lally C, Heath C 1996 Environmental tobacco smoke and coronary heart disease. American Cancer Society. CPS III Cohort (94): 622–628

Stern M P 1995 Diabetes and cardiovascular disease: the 'common soil' hypothesis. Diabetes 44: 369–374

Suadicani P, Heis H O, Gynetelberg F 1993 Are social inequalities as associated with the risk of ischaemic heart disease a result of psychosocial working conditions? Atherosclerosis 101: 165–175

Suadicani P, Hein H O, Gynfelberg F 1997 Weight changes and the risk of ischaemic heart disease for middle-aged and elderly men. An 8-year follow up in the Copenhagen Male Study. Journal of Cardiovascular Risk 4(1): 25–32

Tiefenbrunn A J, Chandra N C, French W J et al for the Second National Registry for Myocardial Infarction (NRMI-2) Investigations 1995 Clinical experience with primary PTCA compared (recombinant tissue-type plasminogen activator) in patients with acute myocardial infarction. Journal of the American College of Cardiology 31(6): 1240–1245

Trials of Hypertensive Prevention Collaborative Research Group 1997 Effects of weight loss and sodium reduction intervention on blood pressure and hypertension incidence in over-weight people with high-normal blood pressure. Archives of Internal Medicine 157: 657–667

Turner R C, Millns H, Neil H A W et al 1998 Risk factors for coronary artery disease in non-insulin dependent diabetes mellitus: United Kingdom Prospective Diabetes Study (UKPDS). British Medical Journal 701: 823–838

VA Coronary Artery Bypass Surgery Co-operative Study Group 1992 Eighteen-year follow up in the Veterans Co-operative Study of Coronary Artery Bypass Surgery for stable angina. Circulation 86: 121–130

Vogh T, Mullooly J, Ernst D et al 1992 Social networks as predictory of ischaemic heart disease, cancer, stroke and hypertension: incidence, survival and mortality. Journal of Clinical Epidemiology 45: 659–666

Watkins P L, Eisler R M, Carpenter L et al 1991 Psychosocial and physiological correlates of male gender role stress among employed adults. Behavioural Medicine 17(2): 86–90

Whetton O K, He J, Cutler J A et al 1997 Effects of oral potassium on blood pressure. Meta-analysis of randomised controlled clinical trials. Journal of the American Medical Association 277: 1624–1632

WHO 1997 World health report. World Health Organization, Geneva

Wong N D, Lupples L A, Ostfeld A M et al 1989 Risk factors for long term coronary prognosis after initial myocardial infarction. The Framingham Study. American Journal of Epidemiology 130(8): 469–480

Yusuf S, Zucker D, Peduzzi P et al 1994 Effect of coronary artery bypass graft surgery on survival: overview of 10-year results from randomised trials by the Coronary Artery Bypass Graft Surgery Trialists Collaboration. Lancet 344: 563–570

8

Men and mental health

Karen Price

If you prick us, do we not bleed? If you tickle us, do we not laugh? If you poison us, do we not die? And if you wrong us, shall we not revenge? If we are like you in the rest, we will resemble you in that.

Shakespeare, *The merchant of Venice*

INTRODUCTION

Mental health was firmly put on the political and health agendas with the publication of *The health of the nation* document in 1991. The White Paper highlighted that 14% of reported days off work are a result of mental health problems and that depression and anxiety alone cost in the region of £6.4 billion a year. These costs are made up not only from the direct costs of consultation and treatment but also the loss of productivity for individuals and carers. It is pertinent that of the 230 per thousand people who go to their general practitioner (GP) with symptoms of a mental illness, only 21 are referred to hospital. A significant number of people are helped in the community. The implication of this is that mental health is a matter of concern for all health professionals, not just the specialist mental health services.

The nature of the differences between men and women continues to cause heated dispute, both in academic circles and in the popular press. This chapter focuses on the fact that there seem to be differences in how men and women appear in the mental illness statistics and that this may have some serious consequences for men. In a chapter devoted to men's mental health and mental illness, it is essential to examine what these concepts mean and where they come from. Without an understanding of the concepts it is impossible to analyse why men are seen to become mentally ill in the way that they do. For this reason I will briefly explore definitions of mental disorder and discuss how, as result of being socially gender constructed, these have a marked impact on how men's mental health needs are identified. These issues will be considered particularly in relation to depression, alcohol misuse and suicide.

MALE AND FEMALE STEREOTYPES

In his chapter on the psychology of sex and gender, Gross (1996) reviews some of the psychological research in this area and introduces the subject by reminding readers of the fact:

that every known culture in the world makes a distinction between male and female, and, in turn, this distinction is accompanied by a widely and deeply held belief that males and females are substantially different as regards psychological make up and behaviour. The particular characteristics and behaviours thought to be typical of males and females in specific cultures are called stereotypes and the study of psychological sex differences is really an attempt to see how accurate these stereotypes are. (p. 574)

That these stereotypes exist is well known. Gross cites the work of Williams & Best (1994) who demonstrated that there is a great deal of consistency across 30 countries in the world about what characteristics are associated with being either male or female or may be seen in both sexes. They did, however, find some variations along cultural lines (see Gross 1996, p. 580; Table 23.1).

Whether there is any truth in these stereotypes, is, however, a different matter. By its very nature a stereotype is based on 'belief' not 'fact'. Gross goes on to cite the large literature review carried out by Macoby & Jacklin (1974) who concluded that many of the stereotypes of male-female differences have little basis in reality. However, Gross also cites Eagly (1983) who believes, on the contrary, that not only is there evidence to support sex differences, but that research has tended to conceal them. This view is further countered by the argument from Macoby (1980) that 'Even if group gender differences are found in a given area of behaviour (physical, cognitive, emotional or social) the differences within each gender are at least as great as the differences between them' (Gross 1996, p. 581).

Bem (1993) identified the schema gender theory, stating that it:

contains two fundamental pre-suppositions about the process of individual gender formation: first, that there are gender lenses embedded in cultural discourse and social practice that are internalized by the developing child, and, second, that once these gender lenses have been internalized, they predispose the child, and later the adult, to construct an identity that is consistent with social conception of gender. (cited in Harris 1995, pp. 138–139).

The acquisition of gender identity certainly starts at birth, if not before. Pleck (1975) makes the point that the construction of gender is not immutable and can be altered by exposure to life experiences, maturation and ageing. 'These late life experiences enrich and loosen one's concep-

Table 8.1 A chronology of masculine gender identity formation (from Harris, 1995)

Level	Stage (age)	Identity formation	Challenging question
Level I Learning how to identify by sex	Early childhood Infancy (0–2) Preschool (2–6)	Unclear Achieving gender constancy Recognition of biological difference	Am I male?
Level II Formation of male gender identity	Primary school (6–12) Adolescence* (12–18)	Key period of formation Reinforce through peers	What is a man?
Level III Trying out identity	Early adulthood* (18–30)	Testing in world	Am I a man among men?
Level IV Affirming identity	Adulthood (30–40)	Form own self-concept	What is most important to me?
Level V Evaluating identity	Maturity (40–50)	The final test	Is this the way I want to be for the rest of my life?
Level VI Accepting identity	Seniority (51–)	Authenticity	Do I like myself?

*These time periods which encompass the years 13–30 will for many men comprise some form of rebellion against father's standards. The vehemence of that rebellion depends upon the quality of the relationship between fathers and sons. The more harsh, judgemental, controlling and punitive a father is, the more angry and rebellious the son will be.

tion of oneself as a man or woman, or they can be occasions of still more distress, discomfort, and feelings of inadequacy' (cited in Harris 1995, p. 173). Thus men's gender identity has the potential to be constantly refined throughout life, though Harris (1995) suggests that at times in the lifecycle some themes predominate, as can be seen in Table 8.1.

The rise of feminism has done much to challenge both men's and women's views of themselves and each other and has been instrumental in bringing about many changes. However, it is important to recognize that while change may bring about opportunities for growth and development, it may also generate a great deal of anxiety. Lloyd & Wood (1996), in their book *What next for men?* have contributions from a number of authors ranging from politicians and poets to academics and journalists. They discuss the kinds of changes that men have been making or trying to resist in the last decades, ranging from the demands made upon men, their role expectations and the effects this has for men and women. One of the contributors, Baker, expresses his concern at the resistance to change demonstrated by phenomena such as the UK Men's Movement, with their agenda to put men back in their 'rightful place' at the head of the table. He suggests that:

The solution is not to reassure men by attempting to halt change, let alone trying to re-create gender relationships now firmly belonging to the past, but rather to help them find new ways of adapting to, and accepting, their emerging new role. This means enabling men not only to come to terms with what they have lost, but also to appreciate how much they stand to gain from adopting a different kind of masculinity. (Baker 1996)

Farrell (1994) also acknowledges the need for men to confront the changes stimulated by feminism, though he questions his past actions in espousing the cause of feminism in the way that he did. He challenges the feminist view that history is men's studies and is critical that this can be used to justify women studying without men. He argues that the belief that this would be 'an attempt to give women something equivalent to what men already have' is not valid. On the contrary, he points out, the patriarchal perspective of the world brings its own problems. 'To a boy, history is pressure to perform ...'.

The view that women *and* men suffer where there is patriarchy is also expressed by Fanning & McKay (1993).

Our society harms men as well as women, in different but equally devastating ways. Men feel an incredible pressure to earn money. Where women are too often considered sex objects, men are just as often considered wage objects or success objects – an equally dehumanising experience.

They go on to challenge the view of women as the only victims and suggest that 'Men are cannon fodder. In all modern wars it is the young men who are expected to leave home, fight, kill and be killed. Society's message to men is that we are expendable'. This is an emotive image but seeks to reframe patriarchy.

In trying to determine what frames male perceptions, Harris (1995) carried out a qualitative piece of research on 560 men in the USA and explored their responses to 24 dominant gender roles. In *Messages men hear*, he suggested that the central thesis for his research is that 'These roles for masculinity are complex, dynamic and contradictory'. He cites Pleck (1976), who distinguishes the demands of the traditional male role (physical strength, impulsive behaviour, display of angry emotions and strong male bonding) from the modern male role (intellectual skills, interpersonal skills, emotional intimacy with women, prohibition of anger, rational control of behaviour and weak male bonding). This underlines the range of adaptation expected of men in recent years. If men are now expected to engage in emotional intimacy with women and be able to express their feelings, though their early socialization has been based on very different demands, then it is hardly surprising that some men will find the transition hard, if not impossible, to make.

This difficulty is highlighted by Formaini (1990) when she says: 'Women speak about their need for intimacy; men talk about their fear of intimacy' (p. 1). As a psychoanalytical therapist, Formaini believes that the demands of masculinity result in men living out their lives 'in a state of isolation from themselves'. This process begins very early in a child's life when a boy is taught that to become a man is to be what a woman is not, a rejection of girlishness, especially of emotional expression. She takes issue with the view of mentally healthy functioning as being centred around the ability to compartmentalize life, where work is work and home is home. It may be functional to society in some ways, as in maintaining profitable work and the status quo, but it carries with it potentially terrible, inhibiting penalties for men.

Formaini feels that the fact that women are the primary carers for children is an important factor in the development of problems for men. This is by no means saying that it is women's fault. She suggests that it is a factor of the developmental process. As children start around the age of 18–24 months to individuate (recognize that they are separate beings from their mothers), it is women who frustrate their wills. 'All children see the woman as the enemy, even though she is also the best-loved one.' As a result of men's distance from child rearing, fathers become a source of 'refuge' from mothers and receive the projection of 'the positive aspects of being human' (p. 41), whilst women receive the projections of all the other experiences. Thus, boys grow up without withdrawing the projections and integrating them into the personality (pp. 47–48).

At this point it may be useful to clarify some terms. To protect the self from anxiety, the mind uses a number of mental or ego defence mechanisms. In psychodynamic theory, these defence mechanisms are *unconscious* ways of trying to deal with conflicts within the human psyche and are used to protect the ego of the individual. Mitchell (1986) points out that: 'There are many things the infantile ego can do by way of protecting itself. It can deny or repudiate unwelcome reality' (p. 20). This is the defence of *denial*. Another primitive defence is that of splitting, where the person splits off unwanted or endangered parts of the self. This is accompanied by projection, pushing the unwanted feelings onto another (Wright 1989, p. 17). The whole process is known as *projective identification*, when the person on the receiving end of the projection starts to take the unwanted feelings into themselves (Spillius 1988, Wright 1989). This can be most clearly seen when mothers become upset when their babies are crying.

What, then, are the consequences for men of this early use of the defences of splitting and projection? If men are split from their feelings, this does not mean that they do not have feelings but that their mechanisms for coping with feelings are limited. Formaini argues that men have learnt that women are potentially dangerous and that they need to ally with other men. This assists the process of identification with what it is to be masculine and fosters ambivalence toward women, since to be male is to reject the feminine and also be unable to reconcile both the love and fear of women. Expression of feelings through the mechanisms used by women is denied to boys and men and their outlet is through potentially 'degraded or sordid means to express distress or unhappiness' (p. 50). Formaini sees that for real change to take place, child rearing should be a truly joint endeavour between parents, which would prevent the destructive use of defences.

That gender is integral to the living of our everyday lives should be clear and Chapter 2 identifies what expectations are placed upon men. These expectations are used to define what is to be considered normal and abnormal and these are concepts central to defining mental health and illness. Yet, in spite of the centrality of gender, Busfield (1996) argues that there is currently no coherent theory for exploring the concept of gender in mental health, since previously offered explanations are inadequate. She argues that gender is 'indirectly embedded in the formal constructions of mental disorder. It is an argument about the construction of categories around gendered feelings, thoughts and behaviours' (p. 103).

DEFINITIONS OF MENTAL DISORDER

Busfield (1996) also argues that a definition of mental disorder is made complex by three key perspectives or 'contested, changing boundaries' (p. 54). The first boundary is that of mental illness. For over a century there has been a process of developing and refining a model of mental disorder as one of psychiatric illness, analogous to physical illness. A number of authors are critical of the way in which what started out as *analogous* has come to be accepted as *identical*. Thus, the study of mental illness has become the proper sphere of expertise for specialist doctors, i.e. psychiatrists, which emphasizes the physical causes and treatments of illness. Critics of the medical model of mental illness condemn the passivity implicit in the model. There is a sense of illness being visited upon one, with little that can be done by the individual to either prevent it or aid recovery.

This view of disorder can be in marked contrast to the second perspective, that of mental disorder as a manifestation of social deviance. A number of theorists have been influential in the development of this perspective. One of the key elements in becoming mentally ill is the process of being so labelled by professionals. This is the view proposed by Scheff (1966, cited in Prior 1993). He argues that there are no clear criteria for diagnosing psychopathology and being labelled as mentally ill is a form of residual deviance: 'That is, deviance which could not otherwise be categorised as criminal or, say, consciously subcultural' (Prior 1993). Prior goes on to point out that 'The idea that mental illnesses were basically forms of social deviance rather than medical disorder had of course been present ever since Parsons (1951) had analysed the compo-nents of the sick role' (p. 139).

Goffman's publications *Asylums* (1961) and *Stigma* (1963) were very critical of the impact of being labelled mentally ill for the individual. The antipsychiatry cry was further developed in the work of Szasz (1970). He also argued the lack of evidence for biochemical disease states in much of psychiatry. He further suggests that the so-called mentally ill who contra-vene society's rules should be seen as deviants and be sanctioned in the same way as any other deviants, not labelled as mentally ill and 'treated'. This is particularly important because we justify all sorts of breaches of individual liberty in the name of psychiatric intervention. Critics of the antipsychiatry view point out that it fails to offer explanations for the emergence of the deviant behaviour and explain the processes that underpin social control (Prior 1993, Pritchard 1995, Busfield 1996).

The third perspective concerns the boundary between mental disorder and mental health. Here, the emphasis is on how we define what is perceived to be normal and what is mental disorder. The concept of normality is by no means a static one and what constitutes normal or mental disorder is subject to review, as evidenced by the changing atti-tudes towards homosexuality, seen by many as no longer a mental illness (Spector 1972).

Adherence to these different perspectives will have a significant impact on the forms of interventions available. These boundaries can be in direct opposition, as when professionals debate over whether a person is mad or bad. The consequence for the individual can be a prison sentence or detention under the Mental Health Act. For health care professionals, there are a number of client problems where the options for intervention are muddied or cynicism takes over. For example, does an individual really want help for their drug abuse problem or do they think it will look good in court and avoid a custodial sentence?

After exploring a variety of explanations of mental disorder, Busfield suggests that it is helpful to consider it in terms of Foucault's representa-tion of madness as the battle between reason and unreason. He discussed this in his work *Madness and civilisation: the history of insanity in the age of reason* (1965). Foucault explored how the mad have moved from being demonized in the Middle Ages to being an 'acknowledged object of scien-tific knowledge' (Kearney 1986). Kearney cites Kurzweil's (1980) discus-sion of Foucault and draws attention to the fact that it is only relatively recently that the mentally ill have been separated from 'thieves and crimi-nals, squanderers and beggars, vagabonds and unemployed. Their sepa-ration from other deviants became a scientific question occupying doctors, lawyers and police' (p. 293).

If designating someone as mentally disordered is based on their perceived unreasonableness or irrationality, it may serve to explain why men, who are thought to be inherently more rational than women, are less likely to be identified as mentally ill. Busfield points out that the polarization of men as rational and scientific and women as irrational and emotional is now well established (see also discussion below on Broverman et al 1970). It may also explain the ambivalence some health care professionals have when working with suicidal patients. If the wish to commit suicide is judged to be the rational choice of a person in intolerable circumstances, then professionals may see intervention from themselves as misplaced paternalism. However, Williams & Morgan (1994) suggest that so-called 'rational suicide' is rare.

It might be argued that with the closure of the large psychiatric hospitals and the loss of beds for the long-term mentally ill, this trend of separating mental illness from other forms of deviance is in danger of being reversed. The Reed Report highlighted the number of mentally ill persons, particularly men, who are being 'cared' for via the prison service rather than psychiatric services. However, there may be a degree to which this is a function of the gender designation of mental illness by the judiciary. 'What is typically problematic amongst men is more likely to be assigned to the category of wrong-doing; amongst women to the category of mental disorder' (Busfield 1996). This does seem to further demonstrate that the differentiation of mental illness and social deviance is by no means clearcut.

'We have to recognise, therefore, that mental disorder is a culturally and socially relative category, whose precise boundaries and meanings vary over time and place and are highly contested. It is, to use the sociological phrase, a "social construct"' (Busfield 1996, p. 59). It is important to note that in spite of manuals on the classification of individual disorders there is still no universally acceptable definition of mental illness.

DIFFERENCES IN ATTITUDES TO MALE AND FEMALE MENTAL DISORDERS

If mental disorder is a social construct and gender is embedded in that construction, then it can hardly be surprising that there are gender differences in the presentation of mental illness (HMSO 1995). When we consider the statistics for admission to psychiatric hospital, it can be seen that more men than women are diagnosed as schizophrenic, alcoholic and drug dependent, that more women are depressed and/or anxious and that more women than men are diagnosed as mentally ill. It is not clear why this should be, especially since it has not always been the case. It is only since the Second World War that men have been the smaller population group in psychiatric hospitals (Lowe & Garret 1956, cited in Cochrane 1983).

How do genders influence the construction of mental health to account for these differences? Cochrane (1983) suggests that:

There are a number of factors in the different roles created by society for men and women, and indeed in the power relationships between the two sexes, which may provide a sounder explanation for sex differences in psychological disturbance. (p. 46)

Broverman et al's (1970) seminal research suggests that there are significant differences in the ways that men's and women's mental health is judged by professionals. The standard for a mentally healthy adult is closely associated with that of a mentally healthy male. Women, however, are seen as more excitable, emotional and less objective and so inherently at a greater distance from what is considered to be a normal mentally healthy adult. Cochrane (1983) cites work carried out by himself and a colleague (Jones & Cochrane 1981) which found that this is the view of the general population as well. 'Thus it may well be that mental illness is seen as essentially a "feminine" quality. In general men are seen to be closer to the general norm of psychological health than women' (Cochrane 1983, p. 49).

There are two contrary positions that can be argued here. If men are closer to the concept of normality, then the statistics would indicate that men are essentially more mentally healthy which, on the surface, seems well and good for men. If, however, the social construction of mental disorder is so distorted by 'the prism of ideology and social interest' (Busfield 1996) then men may be at risk in a number of ways. They may find that their mental health needs are misidentified or completely overlooked. Alternatively, men may feel that they have to cover up their disorder or display it covertly, rather than openly. This in turn may find expression in other deviant forms of behaviour.

DEPRESSION

In considering the diagnosis of depression there are some important questions to ask. First, however, it may be useful to define what is meant by the word depression. This is particularly important because the word has been diluted by its use in everyday life, so that now it is often used as a synonym for feeling fed up or down in the dumps.

Do men get less depressed because they have less to be depressed about? Some authors argue that this is the case, that there are factors in the lives of women that increase the likelihood of depression as a response. As this is a book on men's health, these issues will not be discussed, especially as it has already been done very well elsewhere (see Ussher 1991, Barnes & Maple 1991). However, it is also important to consider other factors that may influence the statistics for men.

Research by Loring & Powell (1988) suggests that even when the symp-

---

Box 8.1 ICD definition of depression

In typical mild, moderate or severe depressive episodes, the patient suffers from lowering of mood, reduction of energy and decrease in activity. Capacity for enjoyment, interest and concentration is reduced and marked tiredness, after even minimum effort, is common. Sleep is usually disturbed and appetite diminished. Self-esteem and self-confidence are almost always reduced and, even in the mild form, some ideas of guilt or worthlessness are often present. The lowered mood varies little from day to day, is unresponsive to circumstances and may be accompanied by so-called 'somatic' symptoms, such as loss of interest and pleasurable feelings, waking in the morning several hours before the usual time, depression worst in the morning, marked psychomotor retardation, agitation, loss of appetite, weight loss and loss of libido. Depending upon the number and severity of the symptoms, a depressive episode may be specified as mild, moderate or severe.

Includes: single episodes of:
- depressive reaction
- psychogenic depression
- reactive depression

Excludes: adjustment disorder (F43.2)
recurrent depressive disorder (F33.-)
when associated with conduct disorders in F91.- (F92.0)

---

toms are equivalent, depression is more likely to be diagnosed in women than in men. However, it is not clear whether this is due to underdiagnosis in men or overdiagnosis in women. Potts et al (1991) suggest that it is a combination of both. They further suggest that there may be several factors influencing this result. First, men may be more likely to deny depression and view it as unproductive and self-indulgent. Second, men are less likely to express their feelings overtly, making it more difficult to detect depression. Third, clinicians do not expect men to discuss their feelings and therefore do not ask about them, which in turn reduces the likelihood of detection (see Potts et al (1991) for the supportive research for these factors). They also found that there were fewer detection errors made by mental health-trained staff.

The implications are important for men. They risk not being identified as being depressed and as a consequence may not be able to gain access to appropriate services for help and treatment. 'This implies that routine depression screening in medical practices may be warranted and that the medical outpatient setting may provide an important opportunity for the recognition and treatment of previously undetected depression, especially among men' (Potts et al 1991). However in the UK the main point of detection is the GP, often the first port of call in health care.

Goldberg & Huxley (1980) identified that the bulk of patients with mental health disorders are dealt with by the primary health care team. They discuss the factors that influence who is identified as having problems and who is not. This demonstrates that the role of the GP is central to patients receiving the support they require and that GPs need to be sufficiently educated to be aware of the difficulties for men.

However, other explanations are posited for the reduced incidence of depression in men that relate to the different roles of men and women. Cochrane (1983) cites the work of Seligman (1975) and suggests that learned helplessness may be a factor in the development of depression. As men are seen to have greater control over their lives, this may be a protective factor in warding off depression. It may also help to explain the increased risk of mental health problems in men as a result of situations where they lose control, as in unemployment (see Chapter 10).

Alongside the issue of control, and the loss of it, is the factor of self-esteem. We are all vulnerable when our self-esteem is threatened or lowered and depression may be a consequence. Jones et al (1995) discuss an interesting area of research exploring whether there is an evolutionary basis for depression, citing Price et al's (1994) claim that 'Depressive states represent a psychobiological response pattern, part of the inherited behavioural repertoire of the human organism'. Jones et al go on to cite Price & Sloman (1987) and Price (1988) who have proposed the hypothesis 'that self-esteem in man is the analogue of resource-holding power in other animals, and loss of the latter is related to low self-esteem' (Jones et al 1995).

Jones et al's research was carried out on male marsupial sugar gliders and whilst it is acknowledged that direct application of animal studies to humans is not possible, their research does give some credence to the fact that lack of access to resources or loss of access, due to being removed from a position of dominance, leads to animal behaviour that can be associated with depression in man. It gives some support to the view that men may be particularly vulnerable when they have experienced loss of self-esteem, be that through divorce, death of a spouse or loss of employment. For those professionals working with men, the detection of risk factors is especially important.

An area where men's self-esteem may be considered to be under attack is where both marriage partners are working and the traditional status of the man's breadwinner role is threatened. Rosenfield (1980) found higher rates of depression in men whose wives were working. However, Cochrane & Stopes-Roe (1980) did not replicate this finding. On the other hand, Glazebrook & Munjas (1986) believe that sex role strain correlates with depression and that changing sex roles are currently increasing role strain for men and women. Although previous research found that women experienced more sex role strain, their study found no difference. 'It is important that therapists assess their assumptions regarding this issue so as not to overlook or minimise the role conflicts of men. Our society widely recognises the conflicts that women face, but only recently recognises the stresses and demands men experience.'

A controversial area of differential rates in mental illness is the marital status of people diagnosed. As both Cochrane (1983) and Busfield (1996) point out, evidence seems to suggest that marriage is a protective factor for men but not for women. There has been considerable debate over why this should be. Aneshensel et al (1981) believe that men benefit from being married and having children at home. Kessler & McRae (1984) suggest that it is not that marriage makes women more depressed but rather there is something in marriage that confers more advantages on men. It may be, as Robertson (1974) suggests, that men are less likely to be admitted to hospital if they have wives able to care for them at home. Some women do seem to take responsibility for their men's health, if they perceive men as not doing it for themselves.

ALCOHOLISM

A key argument put forward by a number of writers is that the incidence of men's depression is lower than that of women because men are more likely to manifest their mental disorder in substance abuse, especially through alcoholism. Whilst alcoholism is not an exclusively male disorder, as previously thought, more males than females are identified as alcoholic. Levin (1995) discusses the disagreements concerning a definition for alcoholism but feels that a most useful description is as follows. Alcoholism is 'drinking more than is good for one over an extended period of time' and incorporates the facts that drinking does serious harm to the drinker, that drinking continues despite its harmful consequences (it is compulsive) and that the harmful drinking continues over a period of time.

A major area of disagreement amongst workers in this field is over what alcoholism is a manifestation of. There are a number of very different beliefs about alcoholism, varying from a form of moral turpitude, a disease or a form of mental illness. Levin's (1995) book provides a very comprehensive discussion of the numerous theories of alcoholism. The research does seem to suggest that alcoholism is a complex area and is likely not to be a unitary diagnosis. Of the various theories available, I will focus on those that may help our understanding of alcoholic men.

Levin argues that one factor in the move towards alcoholism is the pharmacology of alcohol within the human body. Alcohol is a central nervous system depressant. The common misconception that it is a stimulant is a result of the initial response to alcohol at low levels. The individual can experience disinhibition and euphoria as a result of the depression of synaptic transmission. However, the early disinhibition is deceptive as it is followed by depressant activity. The resultant anaesthesia caused by larger amounts of alcohol can be subjectively experienced as a loss of pain. These effects are both illusory and short-lived. Alcohol can get rid of neither depression nor anxiety, as may be the initial feeling. Indeed, the very biochemical nature of alcohol exacerbates both of these conditions and, because of accommodation of the nervous system, demands consumption at greater and greater levels to obtain any relief at all. The terrible paradox results. 'In this respect heavy drinkers drink because they drink. This is truly a case of a dog chasing its tail, a quintessential exercise in futility' (Levin 1995, p. 62).

What would cause a man to start on this 'exercise in futility'? For some theorists the explanation lies in the fact that some people are more susceptible to the demon drink than others. They have an inborn susceptibility to alcohol. Those are the people of whom Alcoholics Anonymous (AA) says: 'One drink is too much, a thousand is not enough'. AA takes the disease approach and this has its positive aspects. It provides a benign explanation that helps to reduce the guilt that is such a feature of alcoholism. Levin points out that AA's heavy reliance on a higher authority (i.e. God) does not fit in with everyone's beliefs. Whilst it may be non-denominational, it is still religious. Critics of the disease theory condemn the passivity inherent in the medicalizing of mental disorder.

To muddy the picture further, not only are there different beliefs about the nature of alcoholism but a number of theorists have identified different types of alcoholism. Winokur et al (1971) defined two types of alcoholism. *Primary alcoholism* is not preceded by any major psychiatric illness, though it may be accompanied by depression. However, the depression will remit with treatment for the alcoholism, especially if the person is able to abstain. Loper et al (1973) found that men have a high depression score on the Minnesota Multiphasic Personality Inventory (MMPI), though this does not persist with recovery. *Secondary alcoholism*, however, follows on from a major psychiatric illness, particularly affective disorders. In this type, alcoholism may be a form of self-medication for the depression and is becoming referred to under the label of dual diagnosis. It is thought that secondary alcoholism is more common in women.

Cloninger (1983) also identifies two types of alcoholism: *male-limited* and *milieu-limited* alcoholism. Whereas *milieu-limited* alcoholism will only become evident if there is an environment to encourage and support it, he suggests that male-limited alcoholism will develop independent of the environment that the man is living in and is characterized by an early onset, severe drinking with inability to abstain, the likelihood of fighting and arrests and little or no guilt about drinking. This form of male alcoholism is similar to the counterdependents identified below. Thus, men are particularly vulnerable because not only are there forms of alcoholism to which they are uniquely vulnerable but the research suggests that they are more at risk of being influenced by alcoholic parents.

Levin cites the work of a number of researchers (Amark 1951, Bleuler 1955; Pitts & Winokur 1966) who have shown that whilst all children of alcoholics are at risk of going on to develop alcoholism themselves, males are at greater risk (p. 121). Goodwin et al (1973) carried out a study of adopted children and found that there was an increased risk of alcoholism in adopted-out sons of alcoholics. Cadoret et al (1984) found adopted-out sons were three times more likely to develop alcoholism.

Cloninger (1983) reports a Swedish study by Bohman (1978). This very large study, based on nearly 1800 adopted-out subjects, found that male-limited alcoholism was nine times more likely in the adopted-out sons of alcoholics. Half the adopted-out sons of male-limited alcoholism became alcoholics (Levin 1995). The fact that there is an increased risk does not confirm clear inheritability but as Levin writes, it does seem to suggest that some form of susceptibility is inherited.

Levin points out that: 'Winokur (1974) has argued that there is a geneti-cally transmitted *depressive spectrum illness* in which women are at risk for depression and men are at risk for alcoholism or sociopathy' (p. 124). Several researchers (MacAndrew & Geertsma 1963, MacAndrew 1965, Hoffman 1973, cited in Levin 1995, p. 125) suggest there is link between alcoholism and sociopathy. They found that there is a raised psychopathic deviate (Pd) scale on the MMPI which may be a measure of the alco-holics' self-reported devil-may-care attitude and an indicator of mild sociopathic behaviour. Thus there is something extremely persistent and characteristic of male alcoholics that is measured by this scale. It is the antecedent of their alcoholism, accompanies it in its active phase and persists with recovery. It is interesting to note that the Pd is raised for women alcoholics yet is not as high as for men.

Men and women seem to respond to the same situation in different ways, as reported by Vance et al (1995). They found that male and female parental responses to perinatal and cot death showed differences, most markedly that women tended to be anxious and depressed more, and for longer, than men. They found that men were more likely to engage in heavy drinking and suggest that 'Increased alcohol use and less psycho-logical distress in fathers may be a manifestation of a different way of coping with such stress. Increased alcohol ingestion in men may also be a way of hiding feelings …'. They feel they have found support for earlier work by Dyegrov (1990) (cited in Vance et al 1995) who also hypothesized that men use different methods of coping and are less likely to acknowl-edge their feelings.

What types of feelings might men have difficulty dealing with? A key issue identified by Formaini is men's difficulty in dealing with their dependency issues. Levin cites the work of Blane (1968) who formulated his theory of alcoholism by working with male alcoholics. He identified three main dependency types. The first type are the dependents, who lack normal healthy interdependence and are openly dependent on others for support. The second type are the counterdependents – their mental defence mechanisms for handling dependence are through denial and reaction formation. Denial has already been discussed above and in this area would be seen when a man is unable to acknowledge his own needs to be dependent. Reaction formation is where a man disguises his needs by behaving in ways that are in opposition to his real needs. The third type are dependent-counterdependents and their conflict around dependency is intense (see Levin 1995, p. 103). Levin argues that from his clinical experience of working with alcoholics, the issue of dependency is centrally important.

Rowan (1997) cites the work of Brannon (1976) who identified four themes of masculinity: *no sissy stuff, the big wheel, the sturdy oak, give 'em hell*. Alcoholism may allow rejection of *the sturdy oak* model and having others dependent on you. The alcoholic male cannot support others when he is incapable of supporting himself. Also, the pressures of being *the big wheel* are lost when the job is lost through drinking. Drinking may also permit externalization of anger that had previously been suppressed. Perhaps through drinking one can partly indulge the expectation of *give 'em hell* without taking the full responsibility for the risk involved.

Whatever the theories for men's drinking suggest, as health professionals we need to move beyond judgement into recognizing that we are working with men in very real distress, who need constructive help, not condemnation. Their problems are not likely to respond easily to intervention but if we fail to identify that those problems exist, then this client group is liable to fall into the last problem area to be considered in this chapter.

SUICIDE

In Britain, suicide is a major cause of mortality, accounting for approximately 1% of deaths. The number of deaths is considered to be significantly higher than this because many suicides are not recorded as such. In 1990, 4485 people killed themselves, something at the rate of 'one person every two hours' (Williams & Morgan 1994). They go on to highlight that whilst the rate of suicide has been growing overall by about 6%, there has been an alarming rise amongst one group: young men aged between 15 and 24. The rate for them rose by 75% in the years between 1982 and 1990. However, the group that is highest over the general average (43% over in 1989) remains the over 75-year-olds. With specific exceptions, such as young Asian women, men are more than twice as likely to kill themselves as women. What are the possible explanations for these statistics?

With the publication of the Government's White Paper *The health of the nation*, suicide has been identified as an area of particular concern. Targets have been set to reduce the incidence of suicide.

To reduce the overall suicide rate by at least 15% by the year 2000 (from 11.1 per 100 000 population in 1990 to no more than 9.4).
To reduce the suicide rate of severely mentally ill people by at least 33% by the year 2000 (from the estimate of 15% in 1990 to no more than 10%).

> **Box 8.2**   Risk factors for depression
>
> - Elderly
> - Male
> - Divorced > widowed > single
> - Unemployed or retired
> - Living alone (socially isolated)
> - Physical illness, especially terminal illness or painful or debilitating illness
> - History of deliberate self-harm
> - Family history of affective (mood) disorder, alcoholism or suicide
> - Bereavement in childhood
> - Social classes I and V
> - Psychiatric and personality disorders

(Adapted from Williams & Morgan 1994)

To assist health care professionals to tackle this issue, the Health Advisory Service published a thematic review entitled *Suicide prevention: the challenge confronted*. As well as assisting in the identification of the risk factors for depression (Box 8.2), a strong message is given that professionals need to challenge their own attitudes towards suicide if they are to be effective in reducing the incidence of preventable suicides.

Williams & Morgan (1994) identify a number of negative attitudes. For example, it is an individual's own choice and decision to commit suicide; once the person has decided to commit suicide you cannot change their mind; people do not seek help if they have decided to kill themselves; until we see changes at the social and political level, there is little chance of having an impact on suicide rates; sometimes suicide is the best solution for a person (pp. 13–16). Negative attitudes can prevent professionals identifying those at risk and becoming actively involved in prevention activities. For this reason, they argue, it is essential that *all* professionals have training in the identification and management of those at risk of suicide.

Farrell (1994) titles one of the chapters in his book: 'The suicide sex. If men have the power why do they commit suicide more?'. He believes that the traditional role of men militates against them seeking help for their problems and argues that men send warning signals but that beliefs about coping and the need to carry on stop them asking for help directly. He further suggests that they fear that an admission of failure will lead to greater failure. The tragedy of suicide is that 'Suicide is the only symptom without chance of a solution' (p. 123).

There is support for Farrell's view that warning signals may have been given out. Vassilas & Morgan (1993) found that 55% of those who had committed suicide had visited their GP in the previous 3 months (cited in Williams & Morgan 1994). This contradicts the view that people who really intend to commit suicide just go out and do it. Williams & Morgan point out that there is considerable ambivalence about taking one's own life and that people '"shop around" for help before killing themselves' (p. 16). The major problem for health care professionals is recognizing what may be the covert cry for help. Therefore, it is critically important that health care professionals are able to recognize the factors that seem to correlate with successful suicide.

It has been argued that one reason more men kill themselves is that they select more lethal methods of suicide. For example, Schwartz & Whitaker found that rates of suicide were lower amongst male students than non-students in the USA, which they attributed as being due to policies that limit access to lethal methods, Pritchard (1995) points out that in Britain, men are more likely to use car exhaust gases or hanging and suffocation, whilst women are more likely to select self-poisoning. Unlike the USA, firearms are the chosen method of a relatively small number of people but men form the highest percentage (5% as opposed to 1% of women). They are most often used by farmers, who are one of the 'at-risk' groups of occupations in terms of suicide. Other occupations include doctors, dentists, vets and pharmacists, who have easy access to methods of self-poisoning. They have the advantage (or disadvantage) of knowing what to take and what constitutes a lethal dose.

If marriage is a protective factor for men's mental health, then the loss of a partner has the potential to be catastrophic. Cattell & Jolley (1995) found that elderly men who commit suicide are more likely to be widowed or separated. A husband whose wife dies is nearly 10 times more likely to commit suicide than a woman whose husband dies (Smith et al 1988, cited by Farrell 1994). Valiant & Blumenthall (1990) suggest that social networks become more resilient as adults develop and social support is a crucial factor in preventing suicide (cited in Winokur & Black 1990). Peaks in suicide rates occur at key points when there is most risk of networks breaking down – adolescence/early adulthood and old age.

However, one of the key causal factors in suicide is mental illness. This is reflected in the *Health of the nation* aims to reduce the rate of suicide in the severely mentally ill. Williams & Morgan (1994) highlight that all mental illnesses carry an increased risk of suicide. In schizophrenia there are some alarming statistics. Miles (1977) suggests that the lifetime risk of suicide is 10%. Of those who commit suicide, 75–90% are male. The first 10 years is the most vulnerable period (Lindelius & Kay 1973, Virkkunen 1974). It is hypothesized that the expectations of the role of men and their difficulty, if not inability, in maintaining these expectations put men under special pressure. Being excluded from the job market traumatizes women less, as traditionally, there is less expectation that they should be the major wage earners.

These factors make it particularly important that health care professionals are vigilant regarding the risk of suicide. If there is a failure to recognize mental illness, then there is a risk of compounding failure to respond to the searching for help. The mythical belief that one can encourage a suicide attempt by talking about a person's intention needs to be exposed as a dangerous falsehood. The intention of more people than is imagined can be established through open and empathic communication on the part of health care professionals (Williams & Morgan 1994).

CONCLUSION

The major theme of this chapter is that while all of us experience risks to our mental health, for men the risk is compounded by the fact that they are not expected to become mentally ill and, if they do, their socialization militates against them seeking the appropriate help. Thus men will require sensitivity in helping them to accept their mental health status and that they have both the need and the permission to do something about it.

REFERENCES

Aneshensel C S, Frerichs R R, Clark V A 1981 Family roles and sex differences in depression. Journal of Health and Social Behaviour 22(4): 379–93

Baker P 1996 Bridging the male crisis. In: Lloyd and Wood (eds) What next for men? London: Working with men

Barnes M, Maple N 1991 Women and mental health; challenging the stereotypes. Venture Press, Birmingham

Bem S 1993 The lenses of gender. Yale University Press, New Haven

Blane H T 1968 The personality of the alcoholic: guises of dependency. Harper and Row, New York

Bohman M 1978 Some genetic aspects of alcoholism and criminality: a population of adoptees. General Archives of Psychiatry 35: 269–276

Brannon R 1976 The male sex role: our culture's blueprint for manhood, what it's done for us lately. In: David D, Brannon R (eds) The forty-nine percent majority: the male sex role

Broverman I K, Broverman D M, Clarkson F E, Rosenkranzt P S, Vogel S R 1970 Sex-role stereotypes and clinical judgements of mental health. Journal of Consulting and Clinical Psychology 34: 1–7

Busfield J 1996 Men, women and madness: understanding gender and mental disorder. Macmillan, Basingstoke

Cadoret R J, O'Gorman T W, Troughton E, Heywood L 1984 Alcoholism and anti-social personality: interrelationships, genetic and environmental factors. Archives of General Psychiatry 42: 161–167

Cattell H, Jolley D J 1995 One hundred cases of suicide in elderly people. British Journal of Psychiatry 166: 451–457

Cloninger C R 1983 Genetic and environmental factors in the development of alcoholism. Journal of Psychiatric Treatment and Evaluation 5: 487–496

Cochrane R 1983 The social creation of mental illness. Longman, Harlow

Cochrane R, Stopes-Roe M 1980 Factors affecting the distribution of psychological symptoms in urban areas of England. Acta Psychiatrica Scandinavica 61: 445–460

Department of Health 1995 Variation in health: What can the Department of Health and the NHS do? London

Dyegrov A 1990 Parental reactions to the loss of an infant child: a review. Scandinavian Journal of Psychology 31: 266–280

Eagly A H 1983 Gender and social influence: a social psychological analysis. American Psychologist

Fanning P, McKay M 1993 Being a man: a guide to the new masculinity. New Harbinger, Oakland

Farrell W 1994 The myth of male power. Fourth Estate, London

Formaini H 1990 Men: the darker continent. Heinemann, London

Foucault M 1965 Madness and civilisation: a history of insanity in the age of reason. Random House, New York

Glazebrook C K, Munjas B A 1986 Sex roles and depression. Journal of Psychosocial Nursing and Mental Health Services. 24(12): 8–12

Goffman E 1961 Asylums: essays on the social situation of mental patients and other inmates. Doubleday, New York

Goffman E 1963 Stigma: notes on the management of spoiled identity. Prentice-Hall, New York

Goldberg D, Huxley P 1980 Mental illness in the community: the pathway to psychiatric care. Tavistock, London

Goodwin D W, Schulsinger F, Hermansen L, Guze S B, Winokur G 1973 Alcohol problems in adoptees raised apart from alcoholic biological parents. Archives of General Psychiatry 28: 283–343

Gross R 1996 Psychology: the science of mind and behaviour, 3rd edn. Hodder and Stoughton, London

Harris M 1995 Messages men hear: constructing masculinities. Taylor and Francis, London

Jones I H, Stoddart D M, Mallick J 1995 Towards a sociobiological model of depression: a marsupial model (Petaurus breviceps). British Journal of Psychiatry 166: 475–479

Jones L, Cochrane R 1981 Stereotypes of mental illness: a test of the labelling hypothesis. International Journal of Social Psychology 27: 99–107

Kearney R 1986 Modern movements in European philosophy. Manchester University Press, Manchester

Kessler R C, McRae J A 1984 Trends in the relationship between sex and psychological distress 1957–1976. American Sociological Review 46: 443–452

Kurzweil E 1980 Michel Foucault: structuralism and the structure of knowledge in the age of structuralism. Columbia University Press, Stanford

Levin J D 1995 Introduction to alcoholism counselling – a bio-psycho-social approach, 2nd edn. Taylor and Francis, Washington

Lindelius R, Kay D W K 1973 Some changes in the pattern of mortality in schizophrenia in Sweden. Acta Psychiatrica Scandinavica 49: 315–323

Lloyd T, Wood T 1996 (eds) What next for men? London: Working with men

Loper R G, Kammeier M L, Hoffman H 1973 MMPI characteristics of college freshmen males who later became alcoholics. Journal of Abnormal Psychology 82: 159–162

Loring M and Powell B 1988 Gender, race and DSM-III: a study of objectivity of psychiatric diagnostic behaviour. Journal of Health and Social Behaviour 29: 1–22

Macoby E E 1980 Social development: psychological growth and the parent–child relationship. Harcourt Brace Jovanovich, New York

Macoby E E, Jacklin C N 1974 The psychology of sex differences. Stanford, CA, Stanford University Press

Miles C P 1977 Conditions predisposing to suicide: a review. Journal of Nervous and Mental Diseases 164: 231–246

Mitchell J (ed) 1986 The selected Melanie Klein. Penguin, Harmondsworth

Pleck J H 1975 Masculinity-femininity paradigm. Sex Roles 1(2): 161–178

Pleck J H 1976 The male sex role: definition, problems and sources of change. Journal of Social Issues. 32: 156–164

Potts M K, Burnam M S, Wells K B 1991 Gender differences in depression detection: a comparison of clinician diagnosis and standardized assessment. Journal of Consulting and Clinical Psychology 3(4): 609–615

Price J 1988 Editorial. Self esteem. Lancet 2: 943–944

Price J, Sloman L 1987 Depression and yielding behaviour: an animal model based on Schjeldering-Elbe's pecking order. Ethology and Sociology. 8: 85–98

Price J, Sloman L, Gardener R J 1994 The social competition hypothesis of depression. British Journal of Psychiatry 164: 309–315

Prior L 1993 The social organisation of mental illness. Sage, London

Pritchard C 1995 Suicide – The ultimate rejection? A psycho-social study. Buckingham, Open University Press

Robertson N C 1974 Relationship between marital status and risk of psychiatric referral. British Journal of Psychiatry. 124: 191–202

Rosenfield S 1980 Sex differences in depression: do women always have higher rates? Journal of Health and Social Behaviour, 21: 33–42

Rowan J 1997 Healing the male psyche: therapy as initiation. Routledge, London

Schwartz A J, Whitaker L C 1990 Suicide among college students: Assessment, treatment and intervention. In: Blumental S J, Kupfer D J (eds) Suicide over the life cycle: Risk factors, assessment and treatment of suicidal patients. Washington D C: American Psychiatric Press, Washington

Seligman M E P 1975 Helplessness: on depression, development and death. W H Freeman, San Francisco

Smith J C, Mercy J A, Conn J M 1988 Marital status and the risk of suicide. American Journal of Public Health 78(1): 79

Spector M 1972 Legitimising homosexuality. Society 14: 52–56

Spillius E B (ed) 1988 Melanie Klein today: developments in theory and practice. Vol 1: Mainly theory. Routledge, London

Szasz T 1970 The myth of mental illness: foundation of a theory of personal conduct. Paladin, London

Ussher J 1991 Women's madness: misogyny or mental illness? Harvester Wheatsheaf, Hemel Hempstead

Vance J C, Boyle F M, Najman J M, Thearle M J 1995 Gender differences in parental psychological distress following perinatal death or sudden infant death syndrome. British Journal of Psychiatry 167: 806–811

Vassilas C A, Morgan H G 1993 General practitioner contact with victims of suicide. British Medical Journal 307: 300–301

Virkkunen M 1974 Suicides in schizophrenia and paranoid psychoses. Acta Psychiatrica Scandinavica. 250: 1–305

Williams J E, Best D L 1994 Cross-cultural views of women and men. In: Lonner W J, Malpas R S (eds) Psychology and culture. Allyn and Bacon, Boston

Williams R, Morgan H G (eds) 1994 Suicide prevention: the challenge confronted (An NHS Health Advisory Service thematic review). HMSO, London

Winokur G 1974 The division of depressive illness into depressive-spectrum disease and pure depressive disease. International Pharmaco-Psychiatry 9: 5–13

Winokur G, Black D W 1990 Suicide and psychiatric diagnosis. In: Blumenthal S J, Kupfer D J (eds) Suicide over the life-cycle: risk factors, assessment, and treatment of suicidal patients. American Psychiatric Press, Washington

Winokur G, Rimmer J, Reich T 1971 Alcoholism IV: is there more than one type of alcoholism? British Journal of Psychiatry 18: 525–531

Wright H 1989 Groupwork: perspectives and practice. Scutari Press, Harrow

9

Men and counselling

Catherine Rhodes

INTRODUCTION

Issues for men as counselling and psychotherapy clients will be examined in this chapter, based initially on an exploration of the development of the male psyche. This frequently affects issues which bring them for counselling, as well as accounting for particular difficulties experienced by men as counselling clients, including their reluctance (when compared with women) to consider counselling to solve or manage problems. Their relationships with a counsellor (or therapist) and the likely effects of gender, of both client and counsellor, on that relationship will be considered.

It is important initially to define the terms 'counselling' and 'psychotherapy'. While there is a plethora of research and writing about counselling for women, there is comparably little on men. In literature searches and reading lists for counselling courses, the topic is grossly under-represented (with the exception of counselling for HIV/AIDS), as compared with that on women. This may reflect the impact of the women's movement in the examination of all aspects of women's lives. Also, it must be acknowledged that far fewer men present for counselling and 'talking' therapies (Relate 1991–4, Maguire 1995); reasons for this may emerge.

WHAT ARE COUNSELLING AND PSYCHOTHERAPY?

Counselling is a growing activity, undertaken in a variety of settings, including counselling and therapeutic agencies, primary and secondary health agencies, the workplace, education (schools, further and higher education), voluntary agencies, specialist and generic settings and the private sector. It is found by many people to offer a safe and supportive environment in which an individual (most commonly, but it may incorporate couples or families) may explore areas of difficulty in their life. Counselling offers a forum where an individual (called hereafter the client) is listened to, supported and challenged non-judgementally. Through this process clients are freed to examine issues, often finding new perspectives or releasing hidden truths on situations, enabling them to live more fulfilled lives (Feltham 1995).

The objectives of particular counselling relationships will vary according to the client's needs. Counselling may be concerned with developmental issues, addressing and resolving specific problems, making decisions, coping with crisis, developing personal insight and knowledge, working through feelings of inner conflict or improving relationships with others. The counsellor's role is to facilitate the client's work in ways which respect the client's values, personal resources and capacity for self-determination. (BAC 1990, p. 3.1)

The focus of this chapter is primarily men in counselling, particularly in the case scenarios. However, a fuller examination of the topic requires consideration of psychotherapy literature. The differences between counselling and psychotherapy are often unclear (Feltham 1995). Both are purposeful approaches in which one person in the role of client (or patient) is helped by another, 'counsellor' or 'psychotherapist', to achieve 'changes in personal functioning' (Aveline 1992). Cawley's model of therapies for the mind defines four levels:

1. support and counselling;
2. psychodynamically focused helping interactions;
3. dynamic psychotherapy;
4. behavioural psychotherapy. (Cawley 1977)

Broadly speaking, differences between counselling and psychotherapy are in therapeutic approach as well as focus, depth of exploration and consequent effect on the client. A medical metaphor could be to compare counselling with a non-invasive medical treatment whereas psychotherapy might be closer to surgery. A client under stress may talk about their difficulties, have their experiences heard and valued and be helped to find better ways of managing this and similar situations; this could be called counselling. An alternative approach might be to examine early infant and childhood experiences and relationships. This helps understanding of how their present reactions were determined in formative years. Through this, they learn that present reactions originate in old psychological defences which are no longer needed; this would be a psychotherapeutic approach. The two processes may achieve a similar effect – the person feels more able to cope and thus feels better, which is the broad aim of all 'talking' therapies. In this chapter, 'counselling' and 'therapy' are used interchangeably, as are 'counsellor' and 'therapist'.

'TELL ME WHERE IT HURTS': DIFFICULTIES PRESENTED BY MEN

The difficulties presented in counselling in one sense are the same irrespective of gender. Counselling involves seeking help for problems in life, with its myriad difficulties for both sexes; complex relationships, grief and loss, illness, sexuality, sexual dysfunction, developmental issues linked to life stages – are all commonly explored. Differences arise in how they are experienced and dealt with by men (Scher et al 1987), not least because men are more reluctant to seek outside help for problems. This is true of physical and psychological difficulties alike.

Some issues are more specific to men. Over recent years, men have felt under assault regarding their male role identity as women's traditional roles have changed, in the aftermath of the growth of the feminist movement. Some men seek help with coping with that perceived threat, others in finding ways to free themselves from stereotypically determined male roles, often through examination of couple or parental relationships and functions. Counselling for redundancy or job threat (euphemistically called 'outplacement counselling') frequently has a larger representation of men than in other types of counselling agencies, from the higher distribution of men in the affected population, especially in senior and middle management positions. The development of counselling for HIV/AIDS has broken new ground in working with grief and life-threatening illness in men, particularly within the gay community.

But what is counselling for? A parallel may be drawn between the application of counselling for psychological distress and pain management. Counselling is concerned with difficulties and distress which cause or carry psychological or emotional pain. If it 'hurts', then counselling may help ease the pain, sometimes offering a 'cure' or possibly alleviating more troublesome symptoms by enabling the person to cope more effectively with their difficulties. Some claim that counselling is only of value for the 'worried well', but for some clients its effectiveness in more serious psychological disturbance has been demonstrated. This includes severe depression and anxiety states, the second and third most frequently occurring mental health problems in the UK (DoH 1993).

Whatever the presenting problem, the focus or nature of counselling may vary. *Crisis counselling* occurs when issues are directly related to the cause of the crisis. This has had high profile recently, being linked to traumatic life events and disasters. Posttraumatic stress disorder is a recognized consequence of life-threatening crisis in which early professional help may help to alleviate longer term disabling effects of accidents, assaults, etc. (Scott & Stradling 1990).

Supportive counselling is the provision of support for a client under pressure from identifiable circumstances which are unchangeable but may continue for a considerable period of time. These are usually deeply distressing 'normal' situations which must be lived through, such as long-term illness or bereavement. Clients are helped to find strategies for coping more effectively and coming to terms with the limitations that their circumstances impose.

Problem-focused counselling refers to issues needing to be worked through to enable a decision to be taken which may lead to action to change the situation. Examples are relationship difficulties, career or employment decisions.

Therapeutic counselling does not necessarily imply a medical model of treatment for a diagnosed condition such as depression, although this might be an appropriate approach. It often focuses on broader existential questions such as the meaning of life, autonomy and death. The essence of this type of counselling is that the therapeutic relationship allows personal growth to occur, which leads to greater self-understanding, personal integration and wholeness.

The focus of counselling will depend partly on what the client wants to achieve and partly on the nature of the problem. Although different categories of counselling focus have been outlined, they are not exclusive and sometimes one presenting problem may lead to another.

Case scenario

A 50-year-old man came for counselling to explore difficulties in his 28-year marriage. In reviewing his relationship with his wife, he decided to end the marriage. In doing so, he found himself challenged by its loss and his own perceived failure of a relationship extending over half of his lifetime. This led him to question what his life had been about. In doing so, he faced the spectre of his mortality, through facing what he called 'mini deaths' in his life, including physical ageing, lost opportunities with his now adult children and a former lover, prospects of winding down to retirement and ultimately fears about his own death. Until he liberated himself from an unsatisfactory relationship and faced his deepest fears, he felt powerless to move forward.

After therapy over a 4-month period, he no longer recognized the man he was. The former man needed to die; he felt that he was starting afresh on a new phase in his life.

MEN AS COUNSELLING CLIENTS: WHY DON'T BIG BOYS CRY?

'Men are taught to apologize for their weaknesses, women for their strengths' (Lois Wise, quoted in Barnett & LaViolette 1993, p. 1). Evidence from the UK and USA shows that counselling and psychotherapy have a far larger female client population, as do mental health services in general

(Scher et al 1987). In agencies offering couple counselling, roughly equal attendance of men and women could potentially be expected. Figures from two UK agencies revealed 16% fewer male than female sessional attendances and 36% more women than men overall. Where couples were seen, twice as many women as men attended (Relate 1991–4, London Marriage Guidance 1994). There are difficulties in identifying figures for one-to-one counselling, but experience would suggest that male-to-female ratios are likely to be considerably lower than that for couples (Bennett 1995). Seeking help from others through talking about emotional difficulties goes against the grain for many men and it may be that men who do come for help are in more serious difficulty than women (Kirschner 1978).

Possible explanations as to why men find counselling less acceptable or more difficult will be explored through examination of psychodynamic developmental perspectives in object relations and analytic feminist and male sex role stereotyping theories. The terms 'psychodynamic' and 'analytic' are used interchangeably in this context as psychodynamic practice is underpinned by psychoanalytic theory (although in practical application in therapy there are significant differences). All these theories are limited in that they seek to explain male sexual difference in white, Western, heterosexual men but fail to address cultural or sexual difference. Developmental theories are similarly limited in examining only children raised in traditional two-parent families.

At the heart of counselling, the client enters into a close but professionally defined relationship with the counsellor in which areas of difficulty may be explored. Being a client involves becoming dependent and vulnerable in an emotionally intimate relationship. It involves willingness to experience potential loss of control and sharing and exploration of uncomfortable feelings. This conflicts directly with commonly portrayed images of masculinity as strong, athletic, successful, decisive, courageous and controlled. Everyday language defines manliness: 'Face it like a man!'. Such stereotypes express ideal manliness, implying what is acceptable or desirable (Fogel et al 1986). What is apparently desirable as a man is to be brave and cope even when life is difficult and fearful. There are few role models for men embodying both masculine and feminine traits but there are many tough images cast in the John Wayne mould. Often, real role models of fathers conform to the traditional male image and, if they do dissent, may be experienced as a disappointment by a son seeking a typecast man on which to model himself. So to turn to someone for help and care is culturally unacceptable. Benjamin (1990) claims that there are elements traceable to boys' early development which make men resistant to the idea of needing or accepting counselling.

Case scenario: The man who couldn't cry

A man in his late 50s was in hospital following mutilating surgery. At first he recovered well, physically and mentally. After being told that he was being moved from the surgical ward to another hospital for rehabilitation, he became acutely depressed, withdrawn and apathetic. Despite the staff's best efforts (including a psychiatric referral), he was unable to talk about his distress. A few days before his planned transfer an inexperienced female worker responded to his distress by putting her arm around his shoulders. He broke down, sobbing uncontrollably. At age 8 he had been given up for adoption by his mother. The last thing he remembered her saying was, 'Come on, you're a big boy now. Be brave for me'. These were the first tears he had shed since, and they started the release of grief pent up throughout his lifetime. This had been made possible by being comforted by a woman with a human gesture, which was what he had needed from his mother. As a child, despite home life being awful, he didn't want to be sent somewhere 'better'. In the hospital, awful things had happened to him, but he did not experience his transfer as progress; it was a reenactment of the loss of his mother and home.

Psychodynamic perspectives

Freudian theory needs to be acknowledged here as the seminal view of male psychological development, although this has largely been superseded by later analytic views (Rayner 1991). Freud identified the key stage in the development of sexual identity in the phallic-Oedipal phase of development (typically between 3 and 5 years). The male child becomes aware of his physical and psychological difference from his mother. Driven by jealousy and in competition with his father for her attention, he desires to replace his father as 'the man' in her life. Because maleness is recognized as being located in the male genitals, Freud postulated that the boy fantasized castrating his father, then as the surviving 'real' or intact man he would replace him. However, because father is the real man and this is a physical impossibility, the boy copes with the uncomfortable feelings by distancing himself from his mother, rejecting her female attributes and identifying more closely with his father. If this phase is successfully negotiated, the boy should develop a mature sexual and personal identity. Once physically fully developed and able to act out sexual desires, memories of love and closeness to the mother remain, but need to be repressed. This repression and distancing from his mother may be expressed in misogyny or in seeking sexual satisfaction without emotional intimacy (Sayers 1986).

Oedipal issues may emerge as difficulties with authority figures, that resemble the father with whom the boy had sought to identify, instead of finding rejection or conflict. They may emerge when issues of counselling supervision (a compulsory requisite of counselling practice) arise.

Case scenario
A male mental health worker who had struggled for many months to express his grief over his mother's death was interrupted by the office window cleaner walking in just as he was about to cry for the first time. He was relieved and, recovering his composure, turned to the counsellor, saying 'That will make for an interesting supervision!'. The female counsellor heard this as 'Just wait 'till Dad hears about this'. To the client, the supervisor represented paternal power and authority over both 'child' and 'mother', in client and counsellor.

Oedipal theory has been criticized in later commentaries as the product of patriarchal ideals, with men perceived as the dominant sex. Indeed, rather than identifying men as the stronger sex, later psychoanalysts suggest that men are psychologically (as well as physically) more insecure and fragile than women. Edley & Weatherall (1995) argue that femininity is the norm from which masculinity deviates. This might explain why far more men than women have conflicts about their sexual identity which may be expressed in transvestism and transsexuality (Stoller 1985, Bland 1993).

Also challenged is the age (in Freudian terms) at which children know they are male or female. Gender identity is now believed to be established at a much younger age, between 18 and 36 months. Most children know their gender and act typically male or female by 2.5 years (Chodorow 1978). This development is affected far more by the impact of external influences (as opposed to innate drives, as proposed by Freud), in particular through close earliest relationships, addressed by object relations and feminist analytic theories. Most men are nurtured for a large part of their early life by a woman as their primary role model (Arcana 1983, Cooper 1986). Even where child care is shared equally, the closely dependent relationship of the early days between mother and infant remains in memory at an unconscious level (Maguire 1995).

Possibly the most difficult transition that a young boy faces is having to adjust perceptions of himself, first away from his mother and then transferred to the father. The developing boy must struggle for sexual identity through acknowledging his difference from his mother, needing to dislocate from identification with her (Greenson 1968). It is suggested that more might 'go wrong' with boys in this complex process. The boy must deny identification with his first major attachment, his mother (there are some parallels here with Freud although the rationale is different), in order to take on the identity of a man. This is at some cost emotionally, which leads to unwillingness to risk closeness and dependence, particularly to a woman, in the same way again. This may go some way to explain why men frequently struggle with intimacy and dependence in relationships, whereas women have more difficulty with loosening attachments and separation from others (Gilligan 1982).

Being in a counselling relationship may mirror the experience of being mothered. Men's fears of entering into this type of relationship again may explain their reluctance to accept counselling — anxiety may be further enhanced because there are more female counsellors than male (Bennett 1995). Also, the reason why separation from identification with the mother occurs is contested. Hudson & Jacot (1991) suggest that this may be biologically driven; by their nature, even when quite young, boys are more active, tolerate frustration poorly, are more aggressive and make less eye contact than girls. As this becomes more marked during his development, so the distance between son and mother increases. Men often criticize the counselling process as being too inactive, having limited structure and direction; this frustrates them and may lead to unsatisfactory outcomes for the therapy (Hunt 1987).

An alternative view is that mothers unconsciously treat boys differently from girls. The baby does not know his gender, but his mother does (Edley & Weatherall 1995). 'As the mother of a son, I recognize the frustration and pain of knowing that my child is at once of my body and alien to it ... Though I made and fed him out of my flesh, I am now "other" than he' (Arcana 1983, p. 1). From birth, different expectations result in a son being communicated with as male. In treating him as masculine, he becomes male (Chodorow 1978). Conversely, a girl is treated as an extension to her mother, in recognition of their sameness.

Missing from both of these theories is the influence of the father as a male role model. In most traditional families there is a triangular relationship of baby–mother–father (Ross 1986). Winnicott (1964), focusing on mother–baby relationships, saw the father's role as passive but vital in supporting the mother–baby unit. But others see that the father's role is proactive in facilitating the boy's disengagement from identification with his mother. In behaving as a man, he provides a role model for the developing boy. Distinctly separate from the mother–child unit, he facilitates the child's ability to differentiate between himself and others. This enables his transition from the close protection of the home to the father's more public world (Edley & Weatherall 1995).

Sometimes difficulties arise as the father (in reality or unconsciously) is experienced by the child as a distant or largely absent figure. Thus the alternative to close mothering is experienced as aloofness or distance in relationships. Another difficulty in identification with the father occurs if he is experienced as weak in relation to the mother, whom young children always see as a powerful figure in their world. If the father is a disappointment, he presents an insubstantial role on which the boy can model himself.

Case scenario

At 30, a man comes for counselling soon after discovering his wife is pregnant. He fears that the child may be a boy, saying he does not know how to be father to a son. He says there would be no problem with a daughter; as the only boy with three sisters, he is far more comfortable with women. Father worked away from home during his early school years. When at home, he was largely uninvolved in family affairs. His mother was critical, involving him in child care only to mete out physical punishment. The client's only involvement with the father had been intermittent discipline, with no balance of care or play. In working through these issues, the client realized how angry he was with his father for being missing throughout his childhood. More predominant was his father's lack of assertiveness, always complying with his mother's restrictive definition of fatherhood. Once his anger and sadness had been owned he was able to create his own more balanced model for being a real Dad to his son. In establishing a good relationship with his son his relationship with his father was able to change, although the sadness remained that it need not have been so.

Sex role theory perspectives

Initially the challenge to the traditional position of men in Western culture has been through perspectives of the feminist movement since the 1970s (Scher et al 1987). At first, it seemed that change was enforced through the identification of men's roles as dominant and, by definition, oppressive to women. So there seemed to be a period of 'male castration'; more recently, it has been recognized that a dominant position in a hierarchy is oppressive and restrictive to those 'on top' as well as those lower in the pecking order.

Challenging traditional stereotypical positions can be liberating for men and women alike. Sex role theory explores the development, attitudes, behaviour and outcomes of traditional and emerging roles for men and women. Therapy may be part of a man's search for answers to the resultant conflicts and dissatisfaction with the traditional male role.

O'Neil (1981) claims that there are two primary outcomes of gender socialization which produce stress and conflict for men: restrictive emotionality and control, and power and competition. While causation and origins of stereotypical roles may be debated, these major outcomes are generally agreed to be encompassed under these headings by sociopsychological and psychoanalytic theories alike. They have consequences for men in their intrapersonal (or internal) world and interpersonal states, affecting home, family, work and career, physical and psychological lives.

Restrictive emotionality is the denial of their own and others' emotional world, resulting in inability to express emotions and/or not allowing others the right to have or discuss feelings. In relationships, talking about feelings is frequently a 'no-go' area. Instrumental reasoning, incorporating logic and rationality, 'has become a common, almost defining characteristic of the male psyche' (Bennett 1995). Vulnerability is unacceptable and may be dealt with by projecting it onto others, including women or 'wimps', or in homophobia. In denying the threat of his own vulnerability, the man is able to feel superior to those thus 'afflicted' and unable to 'cope' (equated with feeling vulnerable). Incongruously, the reverse is closer to the truth, as individuals who repress feelings may make themselves vulnerable to stress-related illnesses including cardiovascular disease and cancer (Cooper et al 1988). Restrictive emotionality is one characteristic of the type A personality (Friedman & Rosenman 1974).

Many men do not have an emotional language; when feelings have been denied and repressed for much of a lifetime, the language with which to express them is underdeveloped. Learning to recognize and identify them may be an essential part of the counselling process for men, but its unfamiliarity and associated anxieties may lead to unconscious sabotage of the counselling, thus avoiding the need to face uncomfortable and unfamiliar feelings.

Case scenario

A middle-aged male client, with a female counsellor, attacked all her attempts encouraging him to connect with his feelings, rubbishing this as 'psychobabble' and intellectualizing about his difficulties. He frequently reiterated that what he wanted were ways to overcome his difficulty, not 'wallowing in emotion'. Paradoxically, what brought him into therapy was his inability to relate to others (particularly women) at anything other than superficial and functional levels and his consequent loneliness. In rare vulnerable moments, he admitted to craving for care and belonging. But the fear of connecting with his feelings and consequent terror of losing control, particularly with a younger woman 'in charge', made him destroy any bid to enable him to find what he desired.

Control, power and competition are defined by O'Neil (1981) thus: 'Control implies to regulate, restrain or to have others or situations under one's command. Power is authority, influence or ascendancy over others. Competition is the act of striving against others to win or gain something'. The three are clearly interdependent, as the need to control self and others feeds the desire to have power and be better than another. There is a splitting of 'good' and 'bad', with strength, power, rationality and success perceived as good and associated with masculinity. Attributes such as intimacy, vulnerability, demonstration of affection, dependency, caring, associated with femininity, are 'bad'. A man may fear being judged as soft, 'sissy' or incompetent by admitting to these. So feminine characteristics essentially threaten the traditional male sex role. This categorization of both roles is limited and may be affected to a greater or lesser degree by factors such as culture, age, class, etc.

The primary goals of male socialization cause role strain. Suffering the stress of role strain, which invokes emotional reactions, further feeds the experience as emotionality, not perceived as an acceptable male attribute, so it is suppressed. When winning is a primary objective, the threat of losing equates with emasculation and failure. In seeking to win all the time, failure is inevitable. For many men, when such a battle is lost, they perceive that they have failed, particularly in a public arena such as work.

Case scenario

A male academic had been a high flyer throughout school, undergraduate and post-graduate years. Now in his mid-40s, despite a senior post in a university department, he came to counselling quite seriously depressed, claiming that he was a total failure. This was based on his perception that he could never be truly successful, as he was not 'good enough' to become a professor. He was a popular tutor with his students, in a successful and mature marriage and was a good and caring father, including sharing care for a disabled son. He denied that these qualities (all based in successful relationships) were important or valuable. His definition of success was in status, money, authority and power. Once he started to explore what this meant, he came to realize that deep down he did not want to go any higher as he really did not want the pressures that this would bring. He had been overwhelmed by fears that, in choosing to stay doing what he was good at, he would be judged by others as incompetent and therefore, by definition, a failure. This had meant he could not enjoy any of his successes or be happy in who he was.

In seeking to attain power and success, others may be treated as objects, as things to be used, not people. Thus interpersonal relationships at home and work may suffer. When the primary goal is winning, interpersonal conflicts may become another arena for competition and a show of strength. The desired outcome is domination over another, not resolution of differences. At an extreme level, this may manifest in abusive relationships. Bennett (1995) suggests that domination and objectification are connected; in identifying another person as an object, they become a thing to be used for the man's own purposes, be that winning, sexual or physical exploitation or psychological domination, thus confirming his identity as a man. Needing to be in control denies other aspects of his character such as caring or vulnerability, which is a loss for himself and others, particularly in relationships. But in objectifying, controlling and dominating, he is as much the victim of gender oppression, in that he cannot allow himself to be weak, vulnerable and cared for.

Case scenario

A young gay man's father was a non-commissioned officer in the army. When together as a family in army houses, he was constantly exhorting his sons to be 'real men', i.e. like him – macho, tough, controlling and competitive. Despite this very real pressure, his younger son realized at an early age that he was different from his peers and how his father wanted him to be. He realized in early adolescence that he was homosexual, eventually coming out as gay at 17, a few months after his father's death. In doing so, he embraced his feminine nature but his father's legacy was that he was fiercely competitive, which extended into his intimate relationships. Unconsciously he sought submissive partners, whom he knew he could beat psychologically. He delighted in belittling them privately and publicly. He came for counselling when he realized that he was having frequent sexual fantasies about wanting to hurt them physically, to prove his domination over them and test their love for him. In exploring this with a male therapist, he acknowledged that he was still trying to please his father. Although he would not deny his sexuality, he could at least be tough in other ways. This proved an impasse as inside there was still a little boy, weak and effeminate in the world of the soldier, but desperate for his father's love.

The deadlock in therapy continued for several months until the day he broke down, realizing how much he had denied that part of himself that wanted to be loved and looked after, wanting to be loved and cared for by his father, but always knowing he would fail him. 'Breaking his heart' (his words) with another man allowed him to relinquish his need to dominate and control and discover that he could express his needs and be shown love in other ways.

GENDER AND THE COUNSELLING RELATIONSHIP

There is limited evidence of the different effects of male–male and female–male therapeutic relationships. Historically, counselling has been mainly practised by women but is based on male orientations from psychology and psychoanalysis. One factor may be the different communication patterns used by men and women, which may determine how same-gender and cross-gender counselling are experienced or understood.

Choice for clients of therapist gender is limited. In the UK, a far greater proportion of trained counsellors are women. This is contrasted by a possibly reversed state of affairs in psychotherapy. So the agency and its orientation determine whether a client will be seen by a male or female therapist; the likelihood of client choice is remote (Bennett 1995).

This has led to feminist criticism of the dominance of men and male approaches in the NHS, where the largest body of users are women, of whom a high proportion state preference for being seen by a woman (Taylor 1991). Similarly, writers on couple counselling have noted a dearth of male counsellors, which may discourage men from attending; where there is conflict in a heterosexual relationship, the man may fear being outnumbered by two women in the counselling room (Chandler

1995). No generic research on male client preferences could be found but, in work with survivors of sexual abuse, 50% of male survivors requested a male therapist. This contrasts with a clear female majority wanting to work with a woman (Walker 1990). Despite the likelihood that most abusers for both groups were men, a higher proportion of men preferred to talk with another man on this issue.

The evidence for men's preferred gender of therapist or of difficulties in therapy between male clients and therapists of either sex is far less clear than is apparently the case for women (Taylor 1991). This is due to varied factors, including lack of direct research. Also needing acknowledgement is that the therapeutic relationship is not determined unilaterally; there are (at least) two in the relationship. Counsellor issues affect their approach and interactions with any client, which stem from their beliefs, attitudes and history, just as they do for clients. It is to be hoped that through training, personal therapy and supervision the counsellor will be self-aware (although in counsellor training the effect of gender is rarely directly addressed). The therapeutic relationship is a result of interaction between two people and the gender of both may be a significant variable in the resultant outcome (other variables include age, marital status, sexual orientation, ethnicity and education).

Whatever the therapist's gender, there is almost always a power differential experienced in a therapeutic relationship, particularly in the early stages. At its simplest, the client has a problem and the counsellor is the helper so dependency and powerlessness are part of the client role. A man's desire for power and control militates against a perceived weaker role in response to someone else, whether male or female. For some men, it may be more acceptable to express weakness and vulnerability to a woman than to another man but for others, the reverse is true. Reaction to therapist gender may be so strong as to determine neither sex of counsellor being acceptable; this reaction is likely to have been determined in earlier relationships.

Men being counselled by a man

Having the common experience of being men together in a specific culture may provide a shortcut in communication. Also, there seem to be differences in the ways that men and women communicate. Having a male counsellor may facilitate more effective communication through use of a common language, often focused on activity and problem solving. It has been suggested that there are higher levels of empathy (vital in effective therapy) between same-sex pairings. However, there are dangers in adhering too closely to this view as identification and empathy are not synonymous.

Empathy requires the counsellor to enter the client's world, putting aside their own experiences and perceptions. The counsellor must hear the *client's* expressed feelings and be able to communicate this understanding effectively to his client, so common experience is not necessarily a prerequisite. When a counsellor identifies too closely with their client's experiences this can cause difficulties; he may assume that he knows what it is like to be this client. However closely matched experiences are, they cannot be the same; each has a unique history. When identification with a client's issues is close, there is always the risk that the counsellor's personal issues, if unresolved, may surface and obstruct effective therapy.

In being counselled by another man, the client might experience deep shame or embarrassment in disclosing his deepest fears and anxieties. This may manifest as hesitancy or outright resistance to the work of counselling. Scher (1987) suggests, however, that a male counsellor who is prepared to be open and accepting of such difficulties may act as a role model for the client to risk greater degrees of openness.

In being close to a man, intimacy and sexual feelings may become confused on the part of client or counsellor. For some men, closeness and sexual expression are inextricably linked and this confusion may tap into homophobic reactions through fear of sexual involvement. This may lead to avoidance of intimacy, counteracting the likelihood of an effective therapeutic outcome. Another difficulty may arise when the counsellor is himself uncomfortable with the open expression of feelings, possibly associating this with loss of control. Where a male therapist's own gender issues are unexplored or unresolved, he may distance himself from male clients psychologically. In doing so, he may perpetuate a client's maladaptive patterns, for example in colluding with intellectualization as a way of avoiding exposing uncomfortable feelings.

Men being counselled by a woman

Carlson (1987) suggests that a man may prefer to have a woman counsellor, fearing humiliation and rejection if he exposes his emotional self to another man. Other men express a feeling of greater safety, with the female role being associated with nurture and care. Having a female therapist may allow exploration of the denied feminine parts of himself (called the 'anima' in Jungian terms (1959), in contrast with his maleness or 'animus'). With a woman acting as counterpart to his view of himself, he may start to experience aspects previously denied, leading to integration of lost parts.

However, therapeutic work for female therapists with men may be far from straightforward. The man may fear that in becoming intimate, he may lose his identity in a smothering, all-engulfing relationship. This may be a recollection (often unconscious) of the struggle to separate from mother, when the alternative to rejecting her is to be engulfed. In entering into an emotionally intimate relationship with a female therapist, these fears may be present, leading to resistance and possible premature ending of therapy. If he allows himself to continue in the relationship, he may discover that intimacy without engulfment and loss of identity is possible.

Fear of expression of difficult emotions may cause the man to become aggressive or seek to dominate the therapist; only when he can feel secure in the knowledge that the direction of counselling is in his control may he relax the struggle and allow himself to enter into a collaborative relationship.

Some men feel that talk about difficult and painful feelings is 'women's work' and so reject encouragement to focus on emotion and their inner life. These differing 'languages' may lead to misunderstanding, where men find difficulty in expressing feelings verbally, wishing to express themselves in focused activity.

There may be an expectation that traditional stereotypical sex roles will continue in the counselling, with the man expecting power and dominance. Unless the woman counsellor resists attempts to 'pigeonhole' her into a deferent role, the therapy is unlikely to proceed effectively for this will reinforce his defences and beliefs about being strong and in charge. A man may be threatened by a woman who challenges him, particularly in the affective arena, where he feels incompetent, and this may result in some form of attack. She needs to remain surefooted but accepting and non-judgemental of his attacks, avoiding defensive retaliation. It is important that the female therapist is sure of her own identity and sexuality to avoid being trapped into stereotyped gender-defined roles in working with men.

Some women counsellors, with a history of abuse by males, may unconsciously wish to 'punish' their male clients, giving them a harder time and showing less empathy than with women. Again, personal awareness, therapy and supervision are vital to protect male clients from such abuse. Some women's experience may have been such that they are unable to work with a man without having a potentially damaging effect on him. For example, a woman who has been abused may find it impossible to 'hear' a man's story, if he has been accused of sexual abuse. Whatever his history, the client has the right to empathic, non-judgemental care. The counsellor must withdraw and refer appropriately, being open that there are difficulties in her own life experience which make working with him impossible.

There may be occasions when a woman is attracted to a male client, maternally or sexually. Maternal or sexual feelings may cause her to protect him inappropriately and, in doing so, she will not challenge him significantly. It is clearly unethical for sexual feeling to be acted out between client and therapist; where this boundary is transgressed, damage to the client is inevitable.

Transference

A frequent occurrence in therapy is the transference of feelings, expected behaviour and qualities which are attributed to the counsellor, although they do not originate there. Their origin is in the client's earlier experiences.

... the patient 'transfers' feelings and attitudes from important figures, especially parental ones, onto the person of the therapist. The patient dresses the therapist, who serves as a manikin, with feelings that have been stripped from others. The relationship with the therapist is a shadow play, reflecting the vicissitudes of a drama that transpired long ago. (Yalom 1980, p. 404)

How transference is used as material to be worked in the therapy depends on the therapist's theoretical orientation. A psychodynamic counsellor would use transferential feelings as raw material for understanding and addressing the client's issues, whereas a person-centred therapist would acknowledge its presence but be less likely to work actively with it.

The relationship between transference and gender is paradoxical; it may occur irrespective of, or be totally determined by, the gender of the counsellor. For example, a female counsellor may be experienced as a father-figure in the client's mind, through their perception of her having power and control in the relationship. Or a male therapist may attract a maternal transference as he is experienced as nurturing and caring. However, the counsellor's gender may be crucial to the work in relation to earlier transferential figures. A request for a therapist of a specific gender may reflect the client's unconscious search to address unresolved issues in relation to that parent (Meyers 1986). Similarly, refusal of a therapist because of their gender may reflect earlier difficulties with someone of that gender. The reactions to and expectations of the therapist may be determined by the client's experience of a parental figure. A client whose parent was cold and critical may respond negatively and with hostility to their therapist. Alternatively, a client may be seeking 'reparenting' by an idealized surrogate parent in the person (or imagined person) of the counsellor, searching for what had been absent in their actual experience.

Case scenario

A middle-aged man came for counselling to examine his deteriorating relationship with his wife. He specifically requested a female counsellor. He was an only child with an absent father and emotionally withholding and critical mother. He married in his late teens, aware he was doing so to escape his mother's influence. On honeymoon, he discovered, however, that his wife was not the kindly accepting person he thought he had married but was, to his horror, a copy of his mother. He tolerated this less than ideal situation for many years, but a life crisis in his early 40s brought him to seek something different. The counsellor was warm and accepted him as he was. Once able to trust that she would not be judgemental, he became strongly attached to her, reenacting differently the relationships with his mother and wife. However, he also had to face disappointment in her being imperfect and unable to fulfil all his needs; at a fundamental level, their relationship was finite and she could not be an all-embracing earth mother for him. Accepting this proved difficult but eventually he could transfer this new experience with a woman outside the counselling room into other relationships.

Because of their development and perceived sex role, men find it hard admitting to or seeking help for emotional distress. Exploring such difficulties through the medium of counselling or psychotherapy is not a natural or ready response for them. However, in the UK, disasters such as Hillsborough, *The Herald of Free Enterprise* and Dunblane exposed raw grief to public gaze. Media coverage, with images of men and women publicly displaying their grief, seriously challenged the need for or rightness of the 'stiff upper lip'. Some men are changing (through free choice or personal or social pressure) and some find that they are able to talk about and reach some resolution of their difficulties in counselling.

REFERENCES

Arcana J 1983 Every mother's son. The role of mothers in the making of men. Women's Press, London

Aveline M 1992 From medicine to psychotherapy. Whurr, London

British Association for Counselling 1990 Code of ethics and practice for counsellors. British Association for Counselling, (BAC) Rugby

Barnett O W, LaViolette A D 1993 It could happen to anyone. Why battered women stay. Sage, Newbury Park

Benjamin J 1990 The bonds of love. Virago, London

Bennett M 1995 Why don't men come to counselling? Some speculative theories. Counselling 6(4): 310–313

Bland J 1993 The dual role transvestite: a unique form of identity. Counselling 4(2): 112–116

Carlson N L 1987 Woman therapist: male client. In: Scher M, Stevens M, Good G, Eichenfeld G A (eds) Handbook of counseling and psychotherapy with men. Sage, Newbury Park

Cawley R H 1977 The teaching of psychotherapy. Association of University Teachers of Psychiatry Newsletter January: 19–36

Chandler K 1995 The company of men. Counselling News 17: 18–19

Chodorow N 1978 The reproduction of mothering: psychoanalysis and the sociology of gender. University of California Press, Berkeley

Cooper A M 1986 What men fear: the facade of castration anxiety. In: Fogel G I, Lane F M, Liebert R S (eds) The psychology of men: psychoanalytic perspectives. Yale University Press, New Haven

Cooper C L, Sloan S J, Williams S 1988 Occupational stress indicator. NFER Nelson, Windsor

DoH 1993 The health of the nation. A strategy for health in England. HMSO, London

Edley N, Weatherall M 1995 Men in perspective: practice, power and identity. Prentice-Hall/Harvester Wheatsheaf, London

Feltham C 1995 What is counselling? Sage, London

Fogel G I, Lane F M, Liebert R S 1986 The psychology of men: psychoanalytic perspectives. Yale University Press, New Haven

Friedman M, Rosenman R H 1974 Type A, your behaviour and your heart. Knopf, New York

Gilligan C 1982 In a different voice. Harvard University Press, Cambridge, Mass

Greenson R 1968 Dis-identifying from mother: its special importance for the boy. International Psychoanalytic Journal 49: 370–374

Hudson L, Jacot B 1991 The way men think. Yale University Press, New Haven

Hunt P A 1987 Marital counselling. Follow-up study of marriage guidance clients: perceptions of the agency, the process and outcomes. Unpublished PhD thesis, University of Aston in Birmingham

Jung C G 1959 Aion. Routledge and Kegan Paul, London

Kirschner L A 1978 Effects of gender on psychotherapy. Comprehensive Psychiatry 19: 79–82

London Marriage Guidance 1994 Annual report. LMG, London

Maguire M 1995 Men, women, passion and power. Gender issues in psychotherapy. Routledge, London

Meyers H 1986 How do women treat men? In: Fogel G I, Lane F M, Liebert R S (eds) The psychology of men: psychoanalytic perspectives. Yale University Press, New Haven

O'Neil J M 1981 Male sex role conflicts, sexism and masculinity: psychological implication for men, women, and the counseling psychologist. Counseling Psychologist 9: 61–80

Rayner E 1991 The independent mind in British psychoanalysis. Free Association Books, London

Relate 1991–4 Statistics from computer databases of five Relate centres (Bristol, Oxford, Northumberland, Cheshire, Sheffield). Relate, Rugby

Ross J M 1986 Beyond the phallic illusion: notes on man's heterosexuality. In: Fogel G I, Lane F M, Liebert R S (eds) The psychology of men: psychoanalytic perspectives. Yale University Press, New Haven

Sayers J 1986 Sexual contradictions: psychology, psychoanalysis and feminism. Tavistock, London

Scher M, Stevens M, Good G, Eichenfeld G A (eds) 1987 Handbook of counseling and psychotherapy with men. Sage, Newbury Park

Scott M, Stradling S 1990 Counselling for post traumatic stress disorder. Sage, London

Stoller R 1985 Presentations of gender. Yale University Press, New Haven

Taylor M 1991 A personal view: how psychoanalysis lost its way in the hands of men: the case for feminist psychotherapy. British Journal of Guidance and Psychotherapy 19(1): 93–103

Walker M 1990 Women in therapy and counselling. Open University Press, Milton Keynes

Winnicott D W 1964 The child, the family and the outside world. Penguin, Harmondsworth

Yalom I D 1980 Existential psychotherapy. Basic Books, New York

10

Men and work

Kevin Mullarkey and John F. Playle

INTRODUCTION

Increasingly, the number of women in employment has grown and this is projected to continue whilst the number of men in employment is likely to continue to fall in the years up to 2006 (Social Trends 1995). This rise in female employment is partly due to the increased availability of part-time jobs, but is also associated with economic and social changes, such as falling birth rates. The economic activity rates for women aged between 25 and 34 years rose by 25% between the years 1971 and 1993, a greater increase than any other group. This may be partly due to a rise in the average age at which women are having children. This suggests that, at least in the middle classes, women are developing their career before having children, indicating a more equal relationship in terms of a career, together with the decision on when and/or whether to have a family. In the same period, the proportion of employed males has decreased in every age group, particularly among men aged 55 and over. The average economic activity rate for men is projected to continue falling in the next 10 years. As a result, women are likely to make up approximately 46% of the civilian labour force in 2006, compared to 44% in 1993 and 37% in 1971.

This chapter considers some of the complex notions and intrinsic natures of the interrelationships between employment, masculinity and health in light of the changing employment situation. Definitions and analysis of the terms 'employment' and 'work' are presented as a basis for discussion of the gendered nature of work. In particular, the centrality of employment to notions of masculinity is examined, including the continuation of the 'breadwinner' role. Recent, present and future demographic statistics are also briefly reviewed in order to consider the consequences and effects that such changing figures may have on future roles and relationships. Some positive and negative effects of both employment and unemployment for men's health are considered. It is concluded that:

- employment continues to be central to an understanding of masculine roles;
- the definition of a single masculinity is problematic;
- while female employment is steadily rising, challenging some previous male roles, perceptions of the traditional male 'breadwinner' role continue as a strong influence on health;
- when considering the complex relationships between employment, masculinity and health, no simple equation can be found;
- employment, unemployment and notions of masculinity affect men's health in positive and negative ways and are only some of the countless psychosocial factors of influence. Employment, however, plays a significant part in defining the more existential purpose for life.

WORK AND EMPLOYMENT AS A CENTRAL FEATURE OF LIFE

What, then, is the motivation for men not only to work, but to invest most of their life energies in gainful employment? George Orwell, writing more than 60 years ago, suggested that:

The truth is, that when a human being is not eating, drinking, sleeping, making love, talking, playing games or merely lounging about – and these things will not fill up a lifetime – he needs work and usually looks for it, though he may not call it work. Life has got to be lived largely in terms of effort. For man is not, as the vulgar hedonists suppose, a walking stomach; he has got a hand, an eye and a brain. (*The road to Wigan pier*, 1937)

Within most contemporary societies it is generally considered that employment, or at least the opportunity to be employed, is a good thing. Indeed, in referring to the five major challenges – or the 'five giants' – evident during the 1930s depression and the subsequent world war, Beveridge (1944) considered the issue of unemployment as 'idleness' – enforced or otherwise. It is not our intention in this chapter to present either a solely negative or positive view of employment in terms of its links to masculinity and health. While Orwell's observations above were made during the depression of the 1930s, the need for fulfilment in life has always been central to our existence. As Orwell suggests, work may be one of the primary ways in which such fulfilment is achieved within society as it is currently organized, although the nature of work has changed in many ways. For men in particular, due to the way in which societal expectations concerning their role as 'breadwinner' have developed, work and, more specifically, employment is often not only a means to fulfilment generally but is in many ways entwined with notions of masculinity; being a 'real man'. It can be argued that ideas about work and being employed have become a key defining feature of masculinity. While such ideas may have changed to some degree, both out of necessity and sometimes desire, the influences of these ideas still permeate men's views of themselves and others' expectations of men (Thomas 1990, Grint 1991). Therefore, the links between ideas about masculinity and the role of employment and unemployment will influence men's health in a number of ways.

The experience of employment differs for individuals; for some, employment may be viewed in negative terms, characterized by low wages, poor working conditions, general exploitation and powerlessness with little job satisfaction. From this perspective, it could be argued that employment in itself may be seen as a threat to general health and well-being. However, for others, the way in which employment offers access to what Jahoda (1982) terms certain 'categories of experience' may be seen as essential to the development and maintenance of general health and well-being. For some individuals, employment may be a positive influence on health, providing more than simply the means to a basic existence. Employment and the nature of work undertaken may be inextricably linked to self-identity, self-esteem and the fulfilment of needs for personal achievement and status.

It is immediately apparent that employment is not a unidimensional concept. Indeed, the nature of employment is multifaceted, not only in terms of its objective features but in the ways that employment is perceived and given meaning by individuals. Whatever the experience of employment for different individuals, Pearson & Reyno (1988) suggest that in most Western societies employment is generally perceived to be preferable to unemployment.

EMPLOYMENT AND WORK: NATURE AND MEANINGS

It is important at this point to explore some possible distinctions between work and employment. Jahoda (1982) suggests that work may be viewed as any activity for a purpose beyond its own execution. Fryer & Ullah (1987) argue that employment, as opposed to work, is not in itself an activity but rather an institutionalized relationship, based most commonly on a contract between an employer and an employee. The selling of labour power for monetary reward is the primary source of existence for most people in current Western society. In this way, individuals provide for and reproduce their material existence, a crucial part of all social existence. The financial income provided by employment is not only necessary for the meeting of basic needs or biological survival; it also becomes a means to other ends – leisure activities, commodity purchases, etc. It is not only the individual in employment who becomes enmeshed in this structure of the wage relationship but also those who are in any way economically dependent upon them. The gendered nature of employment and assumptions about the role of men as providers for family tend to place a great responsibility on men for those seen as dependent on them. This is not to suggest that such assumptions should be accepted uncritically or are not gradually changing, but at a fundamental level it would appear that things have changed little (Morris 1987, Thomas 1990).

However, for the majority of individuals in society, employment is far more than solely an economic matter. It pervades and influences all areas of life – personal, cultural and political. The wider functions or meanings of employment are important. Jahoda (1982) identifies five experiences associated with employment that she sees as linked to the development and maintenance of psychological and social well-being. These are social contacts, status, time structure, activity (physical and/or mental) and having a sense of personal and collective purpose. Fagin & Little (1984, p. 28), summarizing previous literature and research concerning the meanings of work and employment, identify a number of similar broad functions of employment.

- As a source of identity
- As a source of relationships outside the nuclear family
- As a source of obligatory activity
- As an opportunity to develop skills and creativity
- As a factor that structures psychological time
- As a sense of purpose
- As a source of income and control

The extent to which basic differentiations between work and employment are answered by the above explorations is probably negligible. Grint (1991) examines some of the difficulties inherent in trying to clearly define and distinguish between the terms 'work' and 'employment' in more depth and we would direct readers who wish to pursue this conundrum to his work. One way of defining employment may be as any activity which is undertaken for the primary purpose of financial survival. Of course, this is a simplistic definition and one which would receive harsh, well-deserved criticism from sociologists who have made the study of work and employment their task. Clearly, many of Jahoda's 'categories of experience' can be accessed through avenues other than paid employment and most of the purposes of work described by Fagin & Little (1984) may be fulfilled by activities not defined as employment. Despite some of the difficulties in distinguishing between the terms 'employment' and 'work', in the way that Western society is currently organized, employment as one form of work is seen as an essential means to survival, both financially and, it can be argued, psychologically. Pahl (1988) suggests that employment is only one form of work.

Employment as a form of work is one basis on which a state divides the population into those who are 'economically active' and those who are 'economically inactive' (Grint 1991). Even this distinction is problematic when one considers the way in which official statistics relating to employment and unemployment differ dependent upon the definitions of such terms. One of the major ways in which individuals are categorized and describe themselves, beyond those of men and women, is whether they are employed or not. Indeed, if we consider the way in which we converse with others, beyond the initial question of 'Who are we?', the next oft-asked question is 'What do we do?' This can be answered in many ways and were we to dispense with social conventions of meaning, we could reply that we sleep, eat, think, etc., as Orwell acknowledged. However, implicit within such a question is usually the expectation that the individual defines themselves in terms of the nature of their employment (Kumar 1988).

The recognition of employment as a primary source of identity, has been noted by many authors, (Jahoda 1982, Fryer & Ullah 1987, Pearson & Reyno 1988, White 1991). The work that an individual undertakes is often the basis upon which they are categorized, in terms of status, class and influence. Often, it is not only a means of classification of the individual but also of the immediate family, where social class is defined according to the work of the male family member. Many of the family names in Western countries refer to a man's trade or profession by which he was identified, e.g. Carpenter, Smith, Coleman, Seaman.

Today we still generally classify men and women by what they do, rather than other personal characteristics. This is particularly so for men, where assumptions about the value and necessity of paid employment, not only in economic terms, are taken for granted. Whilst for some women an alternative possibility exists in terms of being described as a full-time 'housewife' or 'mother', for men the options are still predominantly those of being employed, unemployed or retired. This is not to say that equal value is placed on the woman's role as full-time 'housewife' or 'mother', but such roles are judged as being more acceptable as an alternative to full-time paid employment.

The high value placed on employment in contemporary society develops from the earliest stages of socialization. The focus of education is primarily oriented towards the goal of employment. Such a high value placed on employment has the obvious corollary of the equally negative value placed on being unemployed. If the status of 'employment' is seen as someone's 'master status' (Goffman 1963), then the devaluing of the state of unemployment may lead to a devaluing of the person who holds that status. Additionally, Goffman's work suggests that there can be similar consequences of the application of such a negative label for those identified with the individual (family and significant others) through a process of secondary stigmatization. In particular with men, the ascription of the 'unemployed' label may undermine a central defining characteristic of their masculinity.

This is not to say that employment is not equally linked to ideas of self-worth for women. Indeed, one of the major criticisms of much of the research and literature on work and employment is that it has been implicitly based on a number of gendered assumptions. Employment has been seen as a male domain, with much of the research consisting of studies of men, by men and from a malestream perspective. Similarly, Marshall (1984) has pointed out that studies of unemployment and its effects have also tended to concentrate on men, based on an assumption that employment is more important to men than women. If one takes such a criticism on board, a fundamental question is raised. This relates to whether, when examining issues of employment and health, gender is seen as the main determining variable for all individuals. Although gender can be seen as one important variable in terms of traditional assumptions about roles, held by society and individuals, a focus on this alone may lead to a narrow analysis of issues, which undermines the influence of other equally significant variables in any proposed relationships. Such other variables would include class, culture and socioeconomic status.

Just as the influence of employment on health may differ dependent on the individual's experiences, so it may be that these experiences will differ according to the nature and conditions of employment. These will inevitably be influenced by other variables such as those highlighted. For the individual in employment who has considerable control and autonomy, finds personal fulfilment, a sense of achievement and reasonable financial remuneration for their efforts, the negative effects of employment on health may be minimal. However, many individuals in employment may have little autonomy, be involved in monotonous work and gain little personal satisfaction and often relatively poor remuneration. For them, work may be seen as a 'necessary evil', simply a means to financial survival and thus contributing little to their health except in terms of being preferable to unemployment. It might be asked whether undertaking any employment is better than none and whether the experience of work and its subsequent impact on health is more influenced by issues such as class than by gender. This is not to deny that gender is important but the complexity of the issue of employment and health must be acknowledged, particularly in light of changing patterns of work and make-up of the workforce.

NOTIONS OF MASCULINITY

Having explored some aspects of the nature and meaning of employment as one form of work, we now turn to the concept of masculinity, before examining the ways in which such a concept links to employment and ultimately to health.

Kimmel (1995) describes the importance of differentiating between sex, i.e. the division of men and women on the basis of biological differences, and gender – '... the cultural meanings that are attributed to such biological differences' (p.viii). This differentiation is of crucial importance in that the biological attributes of being a man are measurable and distinct from those of women. However, when one makes attributions about other characteristics which relate to men and women, one is entering the murky waters of the long-running debates over nature versus nurture. This debate is complex, with a wide variety of views about the extent to which gender identity in terms of certain attitudes, thoughts and behaviours is predetermined by sex (biology) or is socially constructed (created and maintained) through various processes of socialization, conditioning or cultural adaptation (Sabo & Gordon 1995).

Reskin & Padavic (1994) describe gender differentiation as 'referring to social processes that exaggerate the differences between males and females and create new ones where no natural differences occur' (p. 3). Traditional assumptions about the 'naturalness' of certain attributes as belonging to men or women are clearly questionable and although stereotypical images of men and women still exist, many of the fundamental assumptions are rarely accepted uncritically. However, this does not mean that assumptions which underpinned traditional views of gender roles have disappeared or are no longer influential in the organization and division of society.

Notions of masculinity and gender differentiation are of crucial importance, particularly in relation to commonly held beliefs about employment. These gendered beliefs and assumptions are most commonly apparent in arguments about whether employment should be a solely male domain, the nature of employment suited to men and women and the value of employment to men and women. It has been argued that employment is a key factor in the creation and maintenance of gender roles and studies into the experiences of unemployed men seem to suggest that having employment is integrally linked to notions of masculinity – being a 'real man'.

Although changes in the nature of employment, increased unemployment and the higher number of women in the workforce may suggest a reconceptualization of the links between masculinity and employment, evidence from a number of studies does not seem to support any such radical change in position amongst men (Morris 1987, Thomas 1990).

Although the 'facts' may indicate a need for a reconceptualization of 'acceptable' male roles, it would seem that for many men, the concept of the male 'breadwinner' is still alive and well (Morris 1987). The reluctance to relinquish such a view of masculinity cannot be explained solely in terms of the power advantages offered to men by the perpetuation of such traditional views. Such a simplistic argument, though having some validity, fails to acknowledge the ways in which such views are maintained by the wider structures within a society or culture. Lorber (1994) suggests that personal change amongst men will not come about without radical changes in the political, economic and ideological structures which perpetuate and maintain current gender orders.

If, as we have argued so far, gender is a social construction, how do such constructions come about and, maybe more importantly, whose interests do they serve? The question of how gender constructions develop is a bit like the old question of which came first, the chicken or the egg? Does society (whatever that might be) create systems which perpetuate assumptions about gender or are assumptions about gender which are seen as existing 'naturally', through some 'God-given order', merely passively accepted by society? Such allusions to God, however, may in themselves be based on assumptions about the gender of God as both 'Father' and 'Son', ultimate representations of male superiority. Both may contain some element of truth but do not answer the fundamental question. If we take the example of the breadwinner role, do many men accept this role because it is seen as 'right and proper' involving 'different' roles for men and women, and on that basis create and perpetuate systems for employment which express and maintain such roles, i.e. that they are perpetuators of patriarchal systems which maintain a position of power, with the advantages that this may bring?

Alternatively, and somewhat paradoxically, men may also be seen as victims of patriarchy, even if it is created by them, in that hegemonic masculinity may lock them into a position whereby, despite changing trends in employment, there is a lack of opportunity and/or a lack of willingness to redefine the links between employment and masculinity.

One key element to emerge from more recent debates around the study of gender identity, in particular masculinity, is the misguided assumption that a single masculinity exists. Hearn & Morgan (1990) argue that this issue should be considered further because it leads to a naive and reductionist view which reinforces the categorization of all men based on assumptions about 'typical' masculine attributes. Just as gender distinction can be seen as socially constructed and limiting for women, so discussion of a single concept of masculinity denies the importance of difference between men. Indeed, our own views within this chapter, though influenced by theory, also derive from our own experiences, meanings and understandings of being men. Our views and ways of thinking need to be framed within specific contexts. We are both white, middle-class heterosexuals, in rewarding occupations which offer relative autonomy and reasonable financial reward. These can be seen as some of the numerous influences on our masculinities and we would not claim to have access to a global view of a singular concept of masculinity which typifies or unifies all men. We would, in fact, argue that whilst certain characteristics and attributes may be shared amongst different groups of men, the idea of a singular definition of masculinity which treats men as some homogeneous group is ill founded and its limitations need to be acknowledged. However, work and employment continue to be central features of definitions of masculinity at a personal and societal level.

The idea of a labour force, those who work in the employ of others for pay, was largely a consequence of industrialization. The emergence of waged workers led to a distinction between those who worked for pay and those who did not – the employed and the non-employed. However, Reskin & Padavic (1994) argue that this new category of non-employed was problematic in that it did not distinguish between non-workers, such as those who were retired or did not need to work, and those who might be considered unpaid workers. The notion of women as unpaid workers has long been a central theme within feminist debates, in that one of the key aspects related to the value of employment as work rests not upon the nature of work undertaken but whether women are paid for it (Oakley 1985). This unequal relationship between paid and unpaid worker reflects the traditionally functional relationship between the breadwinner and housewife roles, perceived by society to have differing values.

Whilst this chapter is mainly about men, one cannot overlook the unequal system which has traditionally devalued housework, and consequently housewives, and the direct and indirect effects that this may have in terms of an individual's identity. Warr (1982) emphasizes the way in which employment can be seen as vital in contributing to and maintaining a personal identity. Where employment is central to identity, particularly for individual and societal beliefs pertaining to masculinity, then being employed and the nature of that employment can be seen as a crucial factor for the health and well-being of the individual man. Studies amongst men indicate that the loss of employment invariably undermines a man's prior status and has a negative effect on self-esteem and self-image (Shamir 1986, Sheeran & McCarthy 1990). Fagin & Little (1984) identified the experience of unemployment amongst men as frequently characterized by anxiety and distress, often with accompanying signs of depression.

THE CHANGING CONTEXT OF EMPLOYMENT. CHANGING ROLES?

Unemployment is used as both an economic and a social indicator and can be defined in a number of different ways. In the United Kingdom, one method of measuring unemployment is the claimant count, which uses administrative systems to count those people officially signing on as unemployed at government offices. The advantage of this method is that regular statistics are available. However, rules for unemployment and other benefits may be changed from time to time and this affects the claimant count. This method of arriving at unemployment figures attempts to provide a series free from distortions caused by changes in the coverage of the administrative systems. The Employment Department publishes a seasonally adjusted series of figures which is consistent with the current coverage of the count.

In order to fully appreciate the impact of unemployment on men's health, it is necessary to briefly review these figures over the last 20 years and the projected figures for the next 10 years to understand the future trends that may be significant. The number of individuals claiming unemployment benefit rose above the 1 million mark for the first time in recent memory in December 1975 and then to above 2 million in March 1981. The rate of increase then slowed slightly, peaking at 3 million unemployed in February 1985. From the middle of 1986, the number gradually fell to just over 1.5 million in 1990 (arguably after a series of changes to the criteria for inclusion in the figures took place). There was then a sharp rise back up to nearly 3 million in January 1993, since when it has fallen, to just under 2 million in December 1996. The projected figures to 2006 suggest that male employment will fall to 69% actively working (that is, 31% choosing not to work or unable to find work), compared with almost 72% in 1993. Interestingly, during the same period, it is predicted that the figures for females in active employment will increase from 52.6% in 1993 to 56% in the year 2006.

This again demonstrates the changing demography in relation to men's role in the workforce and the potential changes in the inherent nature and purpose of their pursuits and relationships in the future. These figures suggest a more equal platform for both men and women in the future, illustrating the growing possibility of the demise of traditionally ascribed gender roles linked to employment. Clearly these changes will suit some more than others, both men and women.

There is no single consequence of a decreasing male workforce and an increasing female workforce and it would be wrong to assume that there is a simple equation to explain such complex issues within our developing society. There has clearly been a great loss of functions of work, as outlined by Jahoda (1982) and Fagin & Little (1984), with the potential loss of the 'breadwinner' role for many men due to unemployment, amongst other factors. Whilst many women may have found value and purpose in having more freedom and autonomy within their relationship, albeit often born out of necessity, there may be many women as well as men who might prefer a more traditional role. After all, the traditional roles of 'breadwinner' and 'housewife/carer' appear to have offered a great deal of stability and certainty for many individuals, each knowing the expectations as well as limitations of their roles (Davies 1992). There are many working women who, even when the male partner might be unemployed and at home all day, are still expected to fulfil the role of housekeeper, within the traditional boundaries of 'women's work'. This can only be seen as the disadvantage of 'relative freedom', when it is an extra role rather than a developing one, often ending in exhaustion and perhaps additional stress and mental health problems (Pascall 1986).

The stresses and strains may be equal, if different, for the male, who may feel that an enforced role reversal is difficult to accept. Indeed, this has been exacerbated in some more traditional households by these very roles being taken over by the female who has been able to find work. Whilst this is not a new phenomenon, some men may still find this a double loss as one compounds the other. As Cochrane (1983) points out, unemployment is a major determinant of an individual's mental health, especially when 'worklessness' is seen as 'worthlessness'. This negative view can lead to a more serious, downward spiral into mental health problems and psychiatric symptoms.

LOSS OF EMPLOYMENT

Having employment and going to work imposes or provides some structure to life. On a daily basis it provides a routine and it is against the time at work that many other aspects of time are measured, even in their very meaning. The concepts of 'leisure time' or holidays, in essence, relate to time away from employment. The differentiation of time spent in employment and other activities is one of the primary means by which the segmentation and organization of time occurs. Again, as with the orientation to employment discussed above, the imposition of structure upon time commences from early on in life. We are socialized, though some would argue that it is inherent to the human condition, to structure time around more than physiological or biological points such as sleeping, waking, eating, etc. In a much broader time perspective, employment provides some structure to the lifespan. We talk of 'our working lives', retirement from work, etc. These are related to a particular stage of the lifecycle, characterized by employment or employability. This does not mean necessarily that the activities that fill such time in employment are always inherently valued, but the nature of the structuring function seems to serve some purpose and have some value (Jahoda 1982, Fagin & Little 1984).

Employment may have more significant psychological meanings for individuals in terms of being an extension of the person themselves. As has been discussed above, for men this may be particularly true, as the links between concepts of masculinity and having employment still seem central. Employment may meet needs for personal ambition and fulfilment and be a way of channelling both conscious and unconscious drives. At times, this may lead to, or at least be an influencing factor in, the choice of particular occupations and types of employment. In other situations, it may influence the way in which a particular job is undertaken (Ruszcyzinski 1991). The individual's continued drive for maturation and self-fulfilment occurs in two main spheres of life that have the potential to serve in, namely intimate relationships and work activity (Daniell 1985). Obviously, the influence of early experience is important here; how meanings which men attach to work are influenced and learned within the context of the family, education and wider societal beliefs. Meanings then given to work may also link to deeper personal needs being fulfilled. At a fundamental level, employment may provide many individuals with the potential to develop skills and abilities and at times to be creative.

Of course, many of the positive aspects of employment may be provided by other means. However, historically, in particular for men, they have become inextricably linked to current structural forms of employment. Although employment exists primarily for the provision of goods and services mainly for profit, as an unintended, though inevitable consequence it enforces these aspects on all participants. Nowhere else apart from employment are they so linked to a compelling need to earn a living. White (1991) describes how 'Employment is important because it provides income, activity, social contact, and status all in one. As the pivot of modern society, employment also gives cohesion to individuals' lives' (p. 20).

Having discussed the centrality of employment in current society generally, and in particular in definitions of masculinity and the different functions or meanings which employment may have for individuals, it seems appropriate to discuss some of the effects or potential effects of job loss. The initial and in some ways most obvious impact of job loss is the financial hardship or at least the decreased living standards that may ensue. Even amongst those for whom this impact is initially buffered by redundancy payments, it seems likely that some adjustment to loss of income will need to be made. Gordon (1988) suggests that '... the evidence is overwhelming that unemployment causes real financial hardship to those affected' (p. 65) and concludes that all research in this area points to the same conclusion. White (1991) reports that for the vast majority, unemployment generally means that income is cut by at least a half and that financial hardship begins immediately. Reduced income not only affects the abilities of individuals and families to meet 'basic' needs, but may also deny them access to other things such as leisure pursuits, holidays, transport, etc (Morgan & Bradshaw 1987). This may lead to an increased level of isolation, for those who may already be cut off from the social networks that employment provided (Marsden 1982, Fineman 1982).

The direct and indirect consequences for the health of individuals and their families of both reduced income and social isolation are obvious. Some studies have suggested a link between physical ill health and the loss of employment (Fox & Goldblatt 1982, Brenner & Mooney 1983), though the nature and direction of causal relationships has still to be clarified. There is general agreement that unemployment and physical ill health are associated, but other factors such as social class, premorbid states and sustained periods of low standards of living have been identified as contributory (Gordon 1988).

In the case of psychological health and well-being, the research seems to show much clearer correlations between the experience of job loss and negative effects on mental health and psychological functioning (Jahoda 1982, Warr 1982). From the descriptions above regarding the centrality of work and the continued valuing of the 'work ethic' in contemporary society, the impact of job loss, purely from a 'commonsense' point of view, would be presumed to be negative. Warr (1982) emphasizes the way in which employment can be seen as vital in contributing to and maintaining a personal identity.

The ways in which the loss of work invariably undermines individuals' prior status and has a deleterious effect on self-esteem and self-image have been demonstrated (Shamir 1986, Sheeran & McCarthy 1990). Fagin & Little (1984) identified the experience of unemployment as frequently being characterized by anxiety and distress, often with accompanying signs of depression. Job loss not only undermines social status but also invariably brings with it other changes, including disruption in family and work roles, subsequent financial strain, increasing isolation, loss of self-esteem and uncertainty about the future (Jahoda 1982, Ensminger & Celentano 1988). All these factors can have detrimental consequences for psychological health and well-being. Pearlin & Lieberman (1979) identified that the disruptive job events of demotion, being laid off or being sacked had the most profound impact on mental health. They reported that this seemed to be linked to the economic strain and decreased sense of mastery and self-esteem, which were a consequence for the men in their study. Atkinson et al (1986) found that unemployed males in their sample had higher rates of anxiety and depression than employed controls.

It is evident, however, that not all individuals respond to the loss of a job in the same way. Studies have examined variables that may influence and moderate the effects of the experience, some of which are briefly listed below.

- Financial strain (Warr 1982, Payne & Hartley 1987, White 1991)
- Social class/occupational status (Goodchild & Smith 1963, Duff 1982, Warr 1982)
- Length of unemployment (Hill 1977, Jahoda 1982)
- Social support (Warr 1982, Fagin & Little 1984, Atkinson et al 1986)
- Age (Stafford et al 1980, Warr & Jackson 1984)

Findings from these and other studies indicate that the effects of job loss are multidimensional, as are those factors that may influence the subsequent health and well-being of the individual. Discussing a summary of the studies related to job loss and psychological well-being, Liem (1987) concludes: 'They suggest by implication, that working is not simply one of many important factors in emotional health but is a central prerequisite of psychological well-being' (p. 325).

Whilst psychological well-being is covered elsewhere in this book, we need to acknowledge the profound nature of mental distress that unemployment can cause in some individuals. The accompanying sense of loss can initially cause lowered self-esteem, diminished self-respect and feelings of failure (Liem 1987). In some cases this may lead to symptoms of anxiety and mild to moderate clinical depression (Fryer & Ullah 1987). Sometimes the person's feelings of hopelessness can be so profound and the depression so severe that the experience can be likened to a close bereavement, even removing the person's reason and will to live. Ruszczyzinski (1991) even argues that '... the process of mourning may be more difficult to manage after the loss of a job, than after the loss of a loved one' (p. 25). Whereas the lost loved one can never be brought back, in the case of employment, this is usually a possibility. Potential replacement of the lost job exists in reality and in the individual's own hopes. Loss through death is clear – it is irredeemable. With the loss of employment the individual does not know whether it is short term, long term or permanent.

SUICIDE IN YOUNG MEN

The consequences of unemployment for young men are particularly worthy of examination. Studies into the causes of suicide in the 20th century have shown that the dominant factor is a mental disorder and specifically depression (Barraclough & Hughes 1987). The suicide rate is twice as high in men as women and in both sexes the rate rises with age (Sainsbury 1986, Kreitman 1988). Consequently the rate in the 15–24 year age group is usually the lowest figure (Pritchard 1992). In recent years, however, suicide in British men has risen, especially in young men (Burton et al 1990).

Since there is no strong evidence to suggest that mental disorder has increased in this age group (Lehtinen et al 1991), such a significant rise in suicide is probably linked to social factors. Certainly, a number of international studies have made this link (Brenner 1983, Platt 1984, Pritchard 1988) and whilst a causal link is not fully understood, it seems that one influential factor might be the depression and demoralization associated with being jobless (Warr 1987). Such a pressure might be felt more extremely by unemployed young men as they struggle to establish an adult identity. Pritchard (1992) suggests that, with society's demands upon young men with regard to role and achievement, being jobless creates a Durkheimian sense of 'anomie', whereby men are deprived of a central role by virtue of the lack of employment. Whilst Pritchard accepts that a direct causal link between unemployment and suicide is hard to establish conclusively, he nevertheless argues that such a situation, compounded by economic consequences, creates an ethos of hopelessness, which inevitably leads to increased psychological vulnerability.

Due to the spiralling unemployment figures of the last two decades, another group has begun to emerge, namely those who have never experienced employment, a large proportion of whom are men. This new 'underclass', whilst being faced with decreasing opportunities for employment, has at the same time been subjected to a new political culture in which responsibility for self and self-achievement has been the underlying ideology. Whilst many have prospered within this capitalist, New Right economy, for the new emergent underclass, such prosperity may only emphasize the increasing feeling of alienation and disadvantage, as they are unable to share in this supposed success. The longer term effects in terms of health and masculinity of never having worked are still unfolding and as yet uncertain. However, in terms of the masculine role model for children of men who have never worked, there may be concerns about their continued integration into society in order to escape this underclass.

EMPLOYMENT AND STRESS

Most of the evidence discussed so far indicates that the loss of employment is potentially detrimental to men's health. This is not to deny the fact that for some, particularly those trapped in unfulfilling, low-paid and at times hazardous work, employment itself may be seen as detrimental to their health and well-being. This raises the fundamental question of whether any employment is better than none. At times, the loss of employment may be a great relief for some men, especially when their job was a causative factor in developing poor physical or mental health

(Powell & Driscoll 1973, Marsden 1982). However, unless standards of living can be maintained without employment and other purposeful activity can be pursued, the relief from the arduous nature of some forms of employment is likely to be shortlived.

Kornhauser (1985) suggests that mental health in relation to the role of employment is not merely dependent on the absence of specific frustrations but on the extent to which aspects of the work role maintain a realistic, positive belief in oneself and the purposive nature of work activities. He goes on to argue that where the nature of employment is such that it deprives the individual of purpose and 'zest' and leads to negative feelings about himself, poor mental health, characterized by anxieties, tensions, emptiness and a sense of futility, may be an ultimate consequence.

The totally pervasive nature of work within an individual's life means that experiences of stressfulness in employment have potential consequences for the individual's overall health and functioning. We have known for many years that workplace stress imposes a huge cost on the individual, their employing organization and British economy (Cooper & Payne 1988, Cartwright & Cooper 1994). There is much evidence to show how this impacts on the individual's life and whilst these figures are not specifically for men in the workplace, they predominantly refer to men.

Alcohol Concern and the Centre for Health Economics calculate that the costs of alcohol-related problems at work alone are estimated at £72.2 billion per annum in terms of sickness, absence, labour turnover and premature death (Cooper & Earnshaw 1995). Furthermore, the British Heart Foundation Coronary Prevention Group suggests that 180 000 people in the United Kingdom die each year from heart disease (500 people each day) and that heart disease accounts for 70 million lost working days each year to industry and commerce. MIND (1992) claims that 30–40% of all sickness absence from work is attributable to mental or emotional disturbance, some of which is related to stress caused by work. The total national bill for workplace stress is therefore extremely high, estimated by some at 10% of the gross national product per annum (Cartwright & Cooper 1994).

Alexander & Methven (1994) argue that stress at work presents as much of a risk to health as exposure to dangerous chemicals and that employers have a responsibility to protect their employees' mental health. They argue that to do otherwise makes no economic sense, given that stress costs British employers £7 billion and 80 million lost working days per year. The most recent figures (for 1996) suggest that as many as 187 million working days were lost in the UK (CBI 1997), due to stress and low morale.

Whichever of these facts is more accurate, there is undoubtedly an imperative need to consider the effects of employment on men's and women's health. In a decade where 'downsizing' to make an organization more efficient is commonplace, the question of how many staff can realistically be afforded the paradoxical luxury of redundancy, given the need to continue the same or greater rate of output, desperately begs an answer. Whilst the consequences of increased unemployment for those having lost a job have been well documented, the impact on the health and well-being of those remaining in employment is of equal importance. The additional pressures on those remaining in work to work harder for less, along with the constant threat that a climate of potential redundancy poses, may increase the stressfulness of already stressful work.

We need to ask whether, in certain work situations, employment is a price worth paying, given the increased pressures on the remaining workforce. This is in direct opposition to the now famous reply in 1991, by the then Chancellor of the Exchequer, Norman Lamont, on being asked how he might justify the rising unemployment figure. He suggested that unemployment was 'a price well worth paying' in order to keep down the rate of inflation. Given the evidence that has been presented in terms of individuals' experiences of unemployment, or indeed those who were 'fortunate' enough to be kept in work but then still expected to produce as much as when there were more staff, it is difficult to see how the situation could be perceived in such simplistic terms. Rather, just as there is no one single masculinity, neither is there one uniform equation that work equals positive health and that unemployment equals negative health. Neither can the statistics presented here or anywhere else provide the whole picture, for although it is possible to discuss unemployment in terms of varying percentages of the workforce, behind every statistic is an individual or family affected by changing patterns of employment.

Given that the figures outlined above are an accurate prediction, it might be reasonable to assume that there will be more opportunity for men to pursue hobbies and leisure interests in the future. Assuming that individuals are happy with this arrangement and that they have some choice and control over their working and personal lives, this should cause few health problems. However, this again is dependent on the individual's attitude to and view of work. If they only see it as a means to other ends, then there is little problem but if work provides their major social as well as occupational interest, then this may be more problematic, especially if working hours are drastically reduced or, worse, end in redundancy.

Whilst the links between self-concept, being a man and employment remain so closely intertwined and entrenched in current culture, the displacement of employment as central to the concept of masculinity seems a long way off. In a study on long-term unemployed men, White (1985) found that although stressful aspects of a previous job may not have been missed, there was usually a vacuum in the person's life once work was removed. The effects on this group depended on how this vacuum was filled, if at all. The evidence suggested that a positive outlook was maintained by a small minority, about one in eight, who had found something else to give purpose and a meaning to their life in order to feel useful or valued. Access to leisure or alternative activities, however, often depends on resources. White (1991) acknowledges that the long-term unemployed all too often have few material and educational resources and in many instances are also in poorer health than others in employment. He cites the frequent comment about people having the time but not the money, a real challenge to the notion of leisure filling the time that reduced or reducing work creates.

CONCLUSION

In this chapter we have looked at some of the complex issues related to employment, masculinity and health. As well as exploring some definitions of individual terms, we have attempted to examine the relationships which exist between them. The functions of work and employment, beyond merely providing financial income, have been examined. Although we have argued that a single definition of masculinity is problematic, some of the research reviewed here seems to indicate that employment is still a key factor related to masculinities, self-identity and esteem in men.

In light of the changing demography of employment, it might be expected that for men, the somewhat stereotypical role of the male breadwinner may now be outdated. However, whilst some reconceptualization of masculinity and male roles may have taken place, for some men in some circumstances, the research suggests that traditional views and concepts still permeate thinking and actions. If the trends predicted in employment and patterns of work continue, the implications are that the health of men who retain such views may be seriously challenged. It is not only men as individuals who are required to change and adapt, but also the structural aspects of society and culture which perpetuate a view that men's identity and value is to be judged solely by whether they work.

We have explored some of the ways in which both employment and loss of employment may have both positive and negative consequences for men's health. We have only briefly touched on the issue of the new underclass who have never experienced employment and the impact upon their health and well-being in the long term is a subject worthy of follow-up.

The relationship between employment, masculinity and health is complex and cannot be explained separately from the issues of class, culture and poverty. Equally central to an understanding of this relationship is the meanings given to employment by men themselves, which moves the debate beyond the functional definitions outlined by Jahoda (1982) and Fagin & Little (1984). What is apparent, then, is that the experience and nature of employment have the potential to affect men's health in both positive and negative ways.

REFERENCES

Alexander M, Methven S 1994 Hard labour – stress, ill health and hazardous employment practices. Hazard Centres Trust, London

Atkinson T, Liem R, Liem J 1986 The social costs of unemployment: implications for social support. Journal of Health and Social Behaviour 27: 317–331

Barraclough B, Hughes J 1987 Suicide: clinical and epidemiological studies. Croom Helm, Beckenham

Beveridge W 1944 Full employment in a free society. George Allen and Unwin, London

Brenner M H 1983 Mortality and economic instability; detailed analysis for Britain and comparative analysis for selected countries. International Journal of Health Studies 13: 563–620

Brenner M H, Mooney A 1983 Unemployment and health in the context of economic change. Social Science and Medicine 17: 1125–1138

Burton P, Low A, Briggs A 1990 Increasing suicide among young men in England and Wales. British Medical Journal 300: 1695–1697

Cartwright S, Cooper C 1994 No hassle! Taking the stress out of work. Century Business Books, London

Cochrane R 1983 The social creation of mental illness. Longman, London

Confederation of British Industry 1997 Industrial trends survey. CBI, London

Cooper C, Earnshaw J 1995 Corporate liability for stress at work. Journal of Managerial Psychology 10(3): 7–8

Cooper C, Payne R 1988 Causes, coping and consequences of stress at work. John Wiley, Chichester

Daniell D 1985 Love and work: complementary aspects of personal identity. International Journal of Social Economics 12: 48–55

Davies A 1992 Leisure, gender and poverty: working class culture in Salford and Manchester 1900–39. Open University Press, Buckingham

Ensminger M E, Celentano D D 1988 Unemployment and psychiatric distress: social resources and coping. Social Science and Medicine 27: 239–247

Fagin L, Little M 1984 The forsaken families. Penguin, Harmondsworth

Fineman S 1982 White collar unemployment: impact and stress. John Wiley, New York

Fox A, Goldblatt P 1982 Socio-demographic mortality differentials. OPCS series LL No 1. HMSO, London

Fryer D, Ullah P 1987 Unemployed people: social and psychological perspectives. Open University Press, Milton Keynes

Goffman E 1963 Stigma Penguin, Harmondsworth

Goodchild J D, Smith E E 1963 The effects of unemployment as mediated by social status. Sociometry 26: 289–290

Gordon A 1988 The crisis of unemployment. Croom Helm, Kent

Grint K 1991 The sociology of work: an introduction. Polity Press, Cambridge

Hearn J, Morgan D (eds) 1990 Men, masculinities and social theory. Unwin Hyman, London

Hill R 1977 The social and psychological impact of unemployment: a pilot study. Tavistock, London

Jahoda M 1982 Employment and unemployment: a socio-psychological analysis. Cambridge University Press, Cambridge

Kimmel M 1995 Series editor's introduction. In: Sabo D, Gordon D F (eds) Men's health and illness: gender, power and the body. Sage, London

Kornhauser A 1985 The mental health of the industrial worker. John Wiley, New York

Kreitman N 1988 Suicide, age and marital status. Psychological Medicine 18: 121–128

Kumar K 1988 From work to employment and unemployment: the English experience. In: Pahl R E (ed) On work: historical, comparative and theoretical approaches. Basil Blackwell, Oxford

Lehtinen V, Lindholm T, Veijola J 1991 Stability of prevalence of mental disorders in a normal population cohort followed for 16 years. Social Psychiatry and Psychiatric Epidemiology 26: 40–46

Liem R 1987 The psychological costs of unemployment: a comparison of findings and definitions. Social Research 54(2): 319–330

Lorber J 1994 Paradoxes of gender. Yale University Press, New Haven

Marsden D 1982 Workless. Croom Helm, London

Marshall G 1984 On the sociology of women's unemployment, its neglect and significance. Sociological Review 32(2): 234–259

MIND 1992 The MIND survey: stress at work. Employee Counselling Today 4(2): 22–24

Morgan J, Bradshaw J 1987 Budgeting on benefit: the consumption of families on social security. Family Policy Studies Centre, London

Morris L 1987 The no longer working class. New Society 3rd April: 16–18

Oakley A 1985 The sociology of housework, 2nd edn. Basil Blackwell, Oxford

Pahl R E 1988 Introduction. In: Pahl R E (ed) On work: historical, comparative and theoretical approaches. Basil Blackwell, Oxford

Pascall G 1986 Social policy: a feminist analysis. Routledge, London

Payne R, Hartley J 1987 A test of a model for explaining the experience of unemployed men. Journal of Occupational Psychology 60: 228–237

Pearlin L I, Lieberman M A 1979 Social sources of emotional distress. In: Simmons R (ed) Research in community and mental health. JAI Press, Connecticut

Pearson R, Reyno A 1988 Helping the unemployed professional. John Wiley, New York

Platt S 1984 Unemployment and suicidal behaviour: a review of the literature. Social Science and Medicine 19: 93–115

Powell D H, Driscoll S P F 1973 Middle class professionals face unemployment. Society 10(2): 18–26

Pritchard C 1988 Suicide, gender and unemployment in the British Isles and the EEC 1974–85. Social Psychiatry and Psychiatric Epidemiology 23: 85–89

Pritchard C 1992 Is there a link between suicide in young men and unemployment? British Journal of Psychiatry 160: 750–756

Reskin B, Padavic I 1994 Women and men at work. Pine Forge Press, California

Ruszcyzinski S 1991 Unemployment and marriage: the psychological meaning of work. Journal of Social Work Practice 5(1): 19–30

Sabo D, Gordon D F (eds) 1995 Men's health and illness: gender, power and the body. Sage, London

Sainsbury P 1986 The epidemiology of suicide. Williams and Wilkins, New York

Shamir B 1986 Self-esteem and the psychological impact of unemployment. Social Psychiatric Quarterly 49: 61

Sheeran P, McCarthy E 1990 The impact of unemployment upon self-conception: evaluation, affection, consistency and involvement dimensions. Social Behaviour 5(5): 351–359

Social Trends 1995 Central Statistical Office, London

Stafford E M, Jackson P R, Banks M H 1980 Employment, work involvement and mental health in less qualified young people. Journal of Occupational Psychology 53: 291–304

Thomas A 1990 The significance of gender politics in men's accounts of their 'gender identity'. In: Hearn J, Morgan D (eds) Men, masculinities and social theory. Unwin Hyman, London

Warr P 1982 Psychological aspects of employment and unemployment. Psychological Medicine 12: 7–11

Warr P 1987 Work, unemployment and mental health. Oxford University Press, Oxford

Warr P, Jackson P 1984 Men without jobs: some correlates of age and length of unemployment. Journal of Occupational Psychology 57: 77–85

White M 1985 Life stress in long term unemployment. Policy Studies 5: 4

White M 1991 Against unemployment. Policy Studies Institute, London

11

Promoting health to men

Christine Furber

INTRODUCTION

This chapter discusses some of the issues which are important when planning health promotion activities targeting men. These are not intended to be prescriptions for success, but to provide the reader with a basis for reflection and development when introducing such strategies.

There has not been much development of health promotion initiatives for men. This is despite the fact that male life expectancy has been consistently lower than that of women for most of this century and mortality rates of men are greater than those for women (DoH 1993).

Anecdotal evidence suggests that most health promotion activities are directed at preventing diseases and illnesses, such as coronary heart disease and cerebrovascular accidents (stroke), HIV and AIDS, rather than having a direct focus on men and their own health issues. The recent increases in health promotion literature (Naidoo & Wills 1994, Bright 1997) do not reflect the statistics related to men's health. These texts tend to focus on the concepts of health promotion and targets for disease in general, rather than centering on men specifically. However, it is not difficult to find information providing advice and ideas for promoting health to women and children.

Fareed (1994) and Robertson (1995) both suggest that the women's movement of the 1960s contributed to the development of health promotion initiatives directed at women. Fareed suggests that women questioned the services that were available to them and that this, coupled with extended knowledge of their bodies and health, resulted in new services being established. Today, women's health is an accepted part of the health services, with well woman clinics, screening initiatives and self-help groups. However, men's health promotion activities are harder to find.

Robertson (1995) asserts that well man clinics developed during the 1980s with a particular emphasis on screening for illnesses such as cardiovascular disease and diabetes and provision of advice on smoking and diet. He also describes 'sporadic' health promotion activities where services have focused where men gather, such as mobile health promotion units at work places, or advertising about safer sex practices at football grounds. However, he suggests that these are less likely to be accessed by those in lower social groups as evidence from Brown & Lunt (1992) implies that they are mostly attended by those from higher social groups.

MEN'S IDEAS ON HEALTH

Nevertheless, before we consider health promotion and men further, it seems sensible to consider men's understanding of health and the concept of health promotion in general, which has emerged since the late 1980s. Health is a difficult concept to define, mainly because of its subjective nature. In 1946, the World Health Organization defined health as: 'A state of complete physical, mental and social well being and not merely the absence of disease or infirmity' (WHO 1946, p. 1). More recently, many have suggested that this definition is flawed as it does not encompass all the issues which affect health, such as emotional, spiritual and societal factors (Ewles & Simnett 1992) and sexual factors (Aggleton & Homans 1987). Seedhouse (1986) maintains that the definition omits differing value systems and cultural variations in health. These authors see health as a holistic entity affected by many issues.

Some authors choose to describe health from a negative or a positive point of view (Downie et al 1990, Naidoo & Wills 1994). Negative health is the absence of ill health, such as disease, illness or injury. Here, health can be defined from a physical, mental or social stance. In a definition of positive health, well-being is the basic entity. Well-being may be subjective; however, true well-being is described as echoing empowerment where the individual has control of his or her own actions and destiny. For Downie et al (1990), positive health entails true well-being and fitness (strength, stamina, suppleness and skills) within 'an appropriate balance of physical, mental and social ingredients' (p. 23).

Few studies have considered health from a man's perspective. However, in the two that this author has accessed, it is suggested that men view health as a commodity or resource which enables the body to work (Watson 1993, Paxton et al 1994), emphasizing a functional meaning to health. This is consistent with the view of the man as the 'breadwinner' of the family.

Watson's (1993) study of Scottish men also describes health being defined in terms of the body and its relationship to health behaviours, such as smoking, eating and rest. Here, 'healthy' people were defined as those with proportional body weight and height and not excessively indulging in behaviours considered detrimental to health, such as smoking and drinking alcohol. Unhealthy people were defined as those who were grossly overweight and excessively indulged in unhealthy behaviours. Thus, health reflects a balance of body image and healthy behaviour.

Paxton et al's (1994) study of Australian men suggests that men also consider psychological well-being, freedom from illness and psychological fitness as being relevant factors in the concept of health. Again, two-thirds of this study's participants considered behavioural factors and lifestyle issues, such as eating, exercise and smoking, as being causes of illness. These participants also highlighted that environmental issues are relevant, such as pollution and work-related factors.

Despite these studies being conducted with samples from opposite ends of the world (Scotland and Australia), it appears that there are some similarities but also differences in the understanding of health. It follows, then, that it is important when designing health promotion strategies to ascertain the perception of health in the population being targeted, as men are more likely to respond to those which match their opinion of what will be beneficial. Bridgwood et al (1996) recently conducted a survey of adults aged 16–74 years in England which aimed to establish knowledge, attitudes and behaviour towards health. Over three-quarters of men stated that they had 'very good' or 'good' health. Men's views of environmental factors which are bad for their health were mainly pollution, stress and passive smoking, with around half of the respondents citing these. In addition, almost two-thirds consider their own smoking habits and one-fifth their weight, unemployment or alcohol consumption as being health hazards.

Nevertheless, it is important to remember that health care professionals also have their own interpretation of the concept of health and as many of these people have trained within medical paradigms, they may have a negative view of health (Naidoo & Wills 1994).

DEFINITIONS OF HEALTH PROMOTION

The concept of health promotion has become more prominent in the last decade, but the notion first emerged after the World Health Organization's declaration of 'Health for all by the year 2000' in Alma Ata in 1978. Traditionally, the main means of 'health promotion' was using methods to prevent disease and illness, notably health education. However, increasing understanding and development of knowledge of the factors which may affect health have challenged this. Today, there is much debate regarding the meaning of health promotion within relevant literature. The main principles of this are described and the reader is referred to texts at the end of the chapter in order to explore the concept further.

In 1986, the World Health Organization defined health promotion as: 'The process of enabling people to increase control over and to improve their health' (WHO 1986, p. 1) at the first international conference on health promotion in Ottawa, Canada. At the same time, five essential components were also described as being part of health promotion action:

1. healthy public policy
2. creating supportive environments
3. strengthening community action
4. developing personal skills
5. reorienting health services.

Thus, health promotion is seen as being broader than health education alone and encompasses social change (Denny & Jacob 1990).

Health education has historically been criticized because of its 'victim-blaming' approach. Ewles (1993) suggests that it has reflected an authoritarian and paternalistic process as health educators define health needs, and the means of communication, to encourage individuals to change their behaviour. However, this approach, which focuses on disease prevention, has its roots in the medical model which is based on defining the problem causing ill health and then curing this.

As prevention is considered to be better than cure, health education has become the major means used by health professionals to improve health. This approach, though, is narrow, possibly due to its scientific basis. Thus several authors, such as Tones & Tilford (1994), have criticized it for ignoring the effects of socioeconomic disadvantage. However, more recently Tones & Tilford (1994) have explored health education further and now deem empowerment to be a major component. Empowerment is defined as: 'an approach which enables people to identify their own concerns and gain the skills and confidence to act upon them' (Naidoo & Wills 1994, p. 89) and in order to foster empowerment, health education must be a facilitative and enabling process. However, if the individual is to remain in control of their behaviour, they must be assisted to consider their own health needs and to make an informed choice' (Naidoo & Wills 1994, Pike 1995). Rissel (1994) suggests that if the individual has control over their own behaviour, this may facilitate psychological well-being.

Nonetheless, Tones & Tilford (1994) assert that the environment might not be conducive for some to change behaviour due to, for example, poverty but also lack of support. Hence, the importance of healthy public policy has emerged. This means the development of policies which enhance health by making the healthy choices easier; for example, public transport policies providing cheaper and more accessible means of travelling may minimize pollution and stress from driving (Ewles & Simnett 1992).

METHODS OF HEALTH PROMOTION

The term 'health promotion' is often described as an 'umbrella term', embracing a range of methods of promoting health. Health education is only one of these. Healthy public policy which promotes social change through improving living conditions is also involved; areas of action include housing, employment, leisure and equal opportunities (Egger et al 1990, Ewles & Simnett 1992).

Organizational development is an important area where policies which enhance the health of those involved within the organization, for example, healthy catering services, no smoking areas and exercise facilities, are encouraged (Ewles & Simnett 1992). Measures which improve the environment are also considered to be health promoting. Historically, these may have led to clean water and safe sanitation systems, thus minimizing dysentery and cholera. Today, though, these may involve, for example, controlling the use of agents which damage the atmosphere and reduce ultraviolet protection, thus increasing the risk of skin cancer (DoH 1992). Economic and regulatory activities are also included under the health promotion umbrella (Ewles & Simnett 1992). These may involve legislation such as food-labelling regulations, restrictions on cigarette sales to minors and increases in tobacco taxation. Thus, politicians, civil servants and other government officials may become a part of the health-promoting process.

However, individuals may become involved in implementing changes through lobbying and being members of groups. Community development has been advocated as part of the health-promoting process (Ewles & Simnett 1992, Naidoo & Wills 1994). Here, communities are encouraged to work in partnership with health promoters but the community itself identifies its own health needs and develops the confidence and necessary skills to deal with these (Egger et al 1990). Activities in this category involve outreach working (where individuals develop initiatives in the community), networking, encouraging community participants to develop self-help groups, and voluntary groups (Ewles & Simnett 1992). These activities also have the potential to boost positive health through feelings of being in control and enhancing self-esteem (Naidoo & Wills 1994).

Lastly, preventive health services are included in the health-promoting process (Ewles & Simnett 1992). These are seen particularly by doctors as part of the process, due to their medical focus on preventing disease, thus emphasizing negative health. Recently, screening has become an important element of primary health care, focusing on health examinations and blood pressure estimations. Consequently, clinics have developed, such as obesity and smoking, which are linked to the *Health of the nation* targets (Orme & Wright 1996).

From this brief discussion of health promotion, it is apparent that a wide range of agencies may be involved. The concept of 'intersectoral collaboration' is a key principle of the World Health Organization (Delaney 1996). This emphasizes that individuals, groups or communities *work together* with organizations, services or planners in order to promote health. The *Health of the nation* (DoH 1992) strengthened the government's commitment to this through defining the term 'healthy alliances'. The goal of this joint working may be to develop initiatives within community development or healthy public policy.

Many authors are highlighting the benefits of health promotion activities taking place within the context of 'settings' (Naidoo & Wills 1994, Tones & Tilford 1994), also endorsed by the Department of Health (1992). Examples of settings where this may occur are schools, the workplace, hospitals and primary health care.

To conclude, health promotion is a complex process involving a range of methods, activities, individuals and situations. The next section considers how some of these concepts may be used to promote health to men.

SCREENING

Screening has historically been one of the major focuses of health promotion and men. The early well man clinics used this method to identify risk factors in men's lifestyles (Carroll-Williams & Allen 1984, Sadler 1985) and thus tailored advice and interventions to detect and diagnose disease accordingly. Typically, screening methods have detected obesity, hypertension, diabetes, excessive alcohol consumption and smoking complications. More recently, Baker (1996) has described well man clinics which have detected cancers such as prostate and skin, testicular lumps and high blood cholesterol levels which are considered to be a primary cause of heart disease (Francome & Marks 1996).

Since the 1990 General Practitioner Contract was initiated (which encouraged GPs to establish health promotion clinics within the primary health care setting), there has been a proliferation of clinics, particularly related to coronary heart disease, stroke and smoking (Orme & Wright 1996). These clinics are designed to screen for conditions and to help individuals to control these by changing behaviour. Nevertheless, as Orme & Wright suggest, not all GPs have welcomed these opportunities. Some have practical problems of time and resourcing issues, some are concerned about the lack of policies addressing deprivation, while others are concerned because the funding arrangements for initiating these clinics are driving the service.

However, recently concern has also been expressed about the value of such screening methods. The Imperial Cancer Research Fund OXCHECK Study Group's (1994) initial findings suggest that screening, subsequent counselling and follow-up examination and treatment may not be as effective as was initially considered. In particular, blood cholesterol levels in men only reduced by a small amount. Findings from the Family Heart Study Group (1994) also suggest that cardiovascular screening in primary health care is not effective on its own for reducing risk factors in the general population. However, Law et al (1994) highlight that lowering cholesterol levels does have an effect in reducing the risk of heart disease and propose that food should have more detailed labelling so that people have better knowledge of its nutritional content. This would involve healthy public policy methods and include individuals working together from a wide range of perspectives, such as nutritionalists, politicians and food producers. Ralph et al (1996) suggest that men are aware of healthy eating messages, especially those regarding dietary fat, as they were more likely to buy 'low-fat' labelled food than other foods marketed as being 'healthy'. Therefore, 'healthy' food labelling may be a feasible approach in attempts to reduce dietary fat consumption in men.

TESTICULAR SELF-EXAMINATION

Testicular cancer is the commonest form of cancer diagnosed in young men aged 20–34 years in the United Kingdom (Cancer Research Campaign 1991). Many have suggested that testicular self-examination (TSE) is to be recommended for all young men, as this cancer has a high cure rate if detected early (Turner 1995, Cook 1995, Summers 1995, Koshti-Richman 1996). Since the late 1980s, many authors have described TSE and recommended that practice nurses, school nurses and occupational health nurses should be involved in teaching young men to examine their testicles and contact the health services if abnormalities are found (Stanford 1987, Rosella 1994, Turner 1995, Cook 1995, Tugwell 1996). The examination is easy to perform, non-invasive and should be carried out once monthly following a warm bath or shower, when the scrotum is more relaxed. For detailed information on the examination, see Schaufele (1988) or the Imperial Cancer Research Fund's (1995) leaflet 'A whole new ball game. How to check for testicular cancer'.

However, problems with TSE have been documented. Evidence cited by Rosella (1994) implies that few men are aware of the disease, or of TSE. Hence, many suggest that nurses should be more proactive in teaching and promoting the examination. Stanford's (1987) study found that embarrassment was an inhibiting factor for nurses teaching TSE, as four-fifths of the respondents felt that the man would be embarrassed about being taught and three-quarters felt that the nurse would be embarrassed about teaching the examination. Tugwell (1996) states, though, that embarrassment was an issue when she commenced TSE training with army recruits but with more experience, effective use of visual aids and the use of humour in the training session, she felt more comfortable. This suggests that as the trainer develops their expertise, these barriers may be minimized.

Agnew (1996) reported from a British Psychological Society conference and cites evidence from psychologists who recommend that messages regarding screening should be planned to meet the expectations of the target group. Agnew cites Peel (1996) as suggesting that embarrassment was apparent when teenage boys viewed a video of TSE in groups. The boys were interested in acquiring knowledge but wanted to gain information in individual situations, such as using CD ROMs and comic strips, thus using a less formal approach.

Rosella (1994) suggests that there is concern over promoting TSE. Goldbloom (1985) expressed caution over recommending regular TSE to adolescent boys because this might increase their worry and anxiety. He suggests that the examination should be fully evaluated from medical, psychological and financial perspectives before being recommended for all young men.

More recently, Morris (1996a) and Buetow (1996) have questioned the effectiveness of TSE. Buetow (1996) conducted a thorough literature review evaluation of the examination and its suitability as a screening test. He concludes that TSE is not appropriate as a recommendation for all young men, as there is no sound evidence to justify this. He argues that testicular cancer is not a major public health concern as it is still a rare disease and suggests that although TSE itself is an inexpensive and uncomplicated test, all palpable scrotal masses should be viewed with suspicion, thus causing anxiety for those who have false-positive results (Morris 1996a). However, Buetow argues that follow-up tests are costly, thus rendering such screening expensive when compared to the numbers of cancers diagnosed. Buetow also contends that many men delay contacting professionals for advice if a mass is detected, due to fear and embarrassment. Thus, early 'detection' does not necessarily mean early treatment. He also expresses concern that TSE is still rarely carried out by men and that health professionals' commitment to teaching TSE may not be high.

In response to Morris's (1996b) concern over the effectiveness of TSE, Gerrard et al (1996) have recently argued that their TSE programme in primary health care did not increase anxiety; in fact, men were concerned that information regarding testicular cancer was not readily available. However, it is suggested that men with abnormalities of the testicles (namely undescended testicles) are more at risk of developing testicular cancer (Prener et al 1995). Therefore, it seems sensible that these men should be encouraged to perform TSE. Nevertheless, the United Kingdom Testicular Cancer Study Group (1994) suggest that successful correction of this abnormality prior to the age of 10 years may decrease the risk of developing cancer. Thus, the midwife's early detection of any abnormalities, and consequent referral to a paediatrician, is essential after the initial examination of all newborn babies.

It is clear, then, that screening tests should be thoroughly evaluated before they are implemented in order to ensure their effectiveness and appropriateness for all involved. However, as Morris (1996b) suggests, this does not mean that young men should ignore any changes in their testicles; they should develop an awareness of changes in their body and seek professional advice if these arise. Men are often described as not making good use of the health services. However, Bridgwood et al (1996) found that almost two-thirds of all men (compared to almost three-quarters of all women) had consulted a doctor regarding their health in the previous year. This is encouraging, but there are still some groups of men who are hard to reach and community development initiatives are ideal opportunities to meet the needs of those who are particularly vulnerable.

DROP-IN CENTRES

McMillan (1995) describes how a project in Drumchapel, a deprived area of Glasgow, has been established to provide an information and advice 'drop-in' centre for men, but also to provide social support for those with problems of unemployment, isolation and depression. Although men are often described as being reluctant to talk about their feelings, this project has approximately 100 men visiting weekly and a thriving weekly men's group. McMillan explains that one of the reasons for this success is that Tommy Riley, one of its founder members, is a local man who suffered from depression after an illness and being unable to work. However, he became involved in local community issues and consequently, boosted his own self-confidence and self-esteem by developing leadership and negotiating skills. This example demonstrates how becoming involved in community issues can foster empowerment and positive health for an individual. In addition, in being a local man and openly disclosing his own problems, he provides a positive role model and example for those who are willing to help themselves.

Initiatives such as this are increasingly seen to be important in promoting social support and facilitating social networks, especially as there has been a tendency to focus men's health promotion on the individual (Rees et al 1995). Kawachi et al (1996) have recently suggested that social networks, such as having a partner, frequent contacts with family and friends and being involved in church and community organizations, are implicated in reducing the numbers of male deaths from cardiovascular disease, accidents and suicides. Their study also suggested that social networks may extend survival rates after coronary heart disease is diagnosed.

Rowe (1994) suggests that health services for male prostitutes have not been successful in providing acceptable health care or as a means of obtaining information and advice, in order to work safely. He suggests that inflexible clinic opening times, lengthy waiting times and staff disapproval are barriers which inhibit men from attending genitourinary medicine clinics. Rowe explains how the Working Men's Project, based at St Mary's Hospital, Paddington, London, has established a service which provides flexibility, privacy, respect, confidentiality and continuity of carer. Men may telephone to make appointments and then the nurse meets the client in the clinic, hence avoiding embarrassing waiting in public. The client is seen by the nurse who is able to discuss health issues, carry out necessary examinations and initiate treatment if necessary. Thus continuity of carer reduces embarrassment, fosters confidentiality and builds up confidence and trust between client and nurse. However, developing initiatives such as this is hard work. Rowe describes how outreach work and liaison with other agencies was necessary to establish this service and the Project's organizers intend developing this further to include street outreach in pubs and clubs, as well as more formal organizations, such as law courts.

Young men have often been described as a group who are difficult to reach. Bridgwood et al (1996) found that only half of 16–34-year-old men had consulted a doctor in the last year. However, Williams et al (1994) have described how weekly drop-in advice sessions in a deprived council estate have attracted high numbers of young men under 16. The clinic was established to provide family planning advice and contraception to help reduce the unplanned teenage pregnancy rate but a wide range of health advice is also provided. Features which have contributed to this success are convenient, weekly opening times after school and no appointment being necessary. The staff are friendly and cheerful and the same people are involved every week, thus demonstrating a commitment and providing continuity of carer. Flexibility is promoted, as the teenagers may be seen in a group or individually if they prefer. The clinic is also quiet, with no other clinic running simultaneously on the premises. In particular, though, the teenagers are involved in the teaching and encouraged to openly discuss their feelings towards sexual behaviour. Thus, their needs are respected.

HEALTH PROMOTION FOR YOUNG PEOPLE

The Health Education Authority (1996) recently investigated ways of promoting sexual health services to young people (boys and girls) by conducting focus group interviews with 15–21-year-olds throughout England. The young men particularly could not recall any information about family planning services and those that could stated that their friends, peers or family members were the major sources of information and knowledge. Young men also emphasized that family planning services give the impression that they are only for women and that men only attend for free condoms. Davidson (1996) reinforces this, as he states that girls were always the target of sex education in order to prevent unwanted pregnancy. However, Davidson emphasizes that young men do want to talk about sex and explore issues around masculinity. In order to encourage young men to attend family planning services, the Health Education Authority (1996) suggests that the location and means of advertising the service are considered as men are more likely to attend a local service which is inexpensive and will not cause embarrassment.

The Health Education Authority recommend that methods of promoting the service should be variable, but asking young people for their opinions will help to identify the most effective means. They recommend that posters may be used, but that bold, bright colours should be used to highlight key aspects of the service. The words 'sex, free, confidential, private and friendly' must be centrally placed on the poster in order to attract attention. In addition, the words should be large enough to be read from a distance, to avoid embarrassment. Posters should be strategically sited at places frequented by young men, such as sports centres, washrooms of fast food restaurants and cinemas. Leaflets may also be effective. Young men say that photographs emphasizing an informal approach would be helpful and the overall presentation should be non-patronizing and eye catching. As embarrassment was seen to be an inhibiting factor in picking up and reading leaflets, the Health Education Authority suggest that placing them with leaflets which advertised other health issues may improve their uptake.

Davidson (1996) provides sound advice for developing effective sex education with young men. He highlights the need for safety, to facilitate participation. This can be achieved by using small groups and respecting the participants by asking questions and listening carefully. He recommends that, initially, groups should be men only in order to avoid the temptation of trying to impress girls. However, he highlights that mixed-sex groups would be useful later to allow joint discussions. Nevertheless, he explains that the formation of relationships and an understanding of young men's lives are crucial to the success of such discussion groups. Hence, sensitive communication skills are important. He emphasizes that men should be involved with sex education work with young men as this helps to minimize the belief that men are not really interested in this aspect of health education.

HEALTH PROMOTION IN THE WORKPLACE

Several authors promote the advantages of the workplace for initiating and developing health promotion activities (Tones & Tilford 1994, Naidoo & Wills 1994, Griffiths 1996). The workplace is defined by the Workplace Task Force Report (1994) as 'a setting in which renumerative employment is carried out' (Appendix B, p. 1) and provides an example of health promotion activities based on organizational change. This setting has the potential to reach large numbers of healthy men who are otherwise difficult to reach normally (Naidoo & Wills 1994). Health promotion in the workplace has been well established for a while in the USA but only recently have surveys been conducted to investigate the extent of these initiatives in the UK.

The Workplace Task Force Report (1994) found that three-quarters of the workforce and two-fifths of workplaces had access to health education, even though this may be limited, such as using posters and leaflets in some instances. However, the organizations most likely to develop health promotion programmes are those that are larger, have trade unions, belong to the public sector and are owned by overseas-based companies (Workplace Task Force Report 1994, Daykin & Cockshoot 1996).

The Workplace Task Force Report (1994) states that this setting provides access to a wide range of health promotion activities, but smoking policies are the most frequent initiatives, with health education targeting alcohol misuse, nutrition and heart disease the next frequent. The least frequent activities were those which focus on weight control and lifestyle assessment.

Similar findings were reported by Daykin & Cockshoot (1996) in their survey of workplace health promotion in low-paid employment in Bristol. They found that almost three-quarters of organizations had smoking-related activities. However, this survey demonstrated that occupational health initiatives such as risk assessment, accident prevention, eyesight testing and back care are also more common than lifestyle interventions.

Both surveys suggest that the use of posters and leaflets to educate about health issues appears to be very common in the workplace. However, regarding smoking interventions, the main focus seems to be banning, or partially banning, smoking on the premises. Reid et al (1992) suggest that bans on smoking in public places may be more effective as 'supporting measures', with interventions focusing on the individual being used as well. Nevertheless, the surveys did find that around one-fifth of organizations do provide smoking cessation counselling.

The workplace is a particularly good setting in which to promote the area of mental health. As Bridgwood et al (1996) state that over half of the men in their survey had experienced a 'large' or 'moderate' amount of stress in the previous 12 months, stress is a significant health issue. The Workplace Task Force Report (1994) suggests that stress can be reduced by recognizing and minimizing stressors within the workplace itself, but also by employing stress management programmes and providing support for employees. They also advise that this setting has the potential to decrease the stigma attached to mental health problems.

Daykin & Cockshoot (1996) found that nearly two-fifths of employers facilitated flexible work breaks to help minimize stress, whilst one-third used organizational changes such as more effective communication methods to deal with this. Stress management training and counselling was also used by one-third of employers. Naidoo & Wills (1994) suggest that the workplace itself can be harmful through generating stress, whilst Johnson et al (1996) have recently found that men who have minimal control over their work have a greater risk of developing cardiovascular disease. Hence, employers should regularly monitor stress levels within the organization to identify risk factors and make changes to minimize these (Workplace Task Force Report 1994).

The workplace may also provide the opportunity to identify those who may be at risk of worsening mental health or even harming themselves, as Chooramun & Phee (1997) suggest that mental health problems may initially emerge here. Thus, facilitating support or referral for medical help may be appropriate. The Workplace Task Force Report (1994) also suggests that rehabilitation programmes which are sensitive to the individual's needs and abilities will help facilitate a successful return to work. Thus, liaison between the employee, manager and health professionals is important.

Naidoo & Wills (1994) have criticized workplace health promotion strategies for their tendency to focus on the individual and overlook organizational and environmental interventions. However, Sorensen et al (1996) have recently described how preliminary results from the Working Well Trial in America have demonstrated that a nutrition intervention has resulted in small but significant reductions in fat consumption and increases of fruit and vegetable intake. This intervention was comprehensive and involved an individual focus using posters, leaflets, self-help materials, self-assessments and education through groups, but also organizational change through catering policies and changes in food available in cafeterias and vending machines.

North American, Scandinavian and Japanese evidence on the effectiveness of workplace health promotion demonstrates that comprehensive programmes addressing the work environment, mental health and stress minimization and lifestyle changes are more likely to be successful (Simnett 1995). Those which target the individual only, such as screening, are less likely to have positive health benefits. Simnett also suggests that those interventions which the employees themselves help to develop have more chance of success. Daykin & Cockshoot (1996) found that almost one-third of respondents in their survey did not involve workers in planning health promotion activities, although consultation did occur in one-quarter of respondents. Their survey also highlighted that over half of the responding organizations had personnel managers involved in planning initiatives. However, the authors suggest that management involvement in health promotion might deter some low-paid workers from participating due to fears that information about their health may be used against them if jobs are under threat.

HEALTH PROMOTION IN SCHOOLS

Another setting which has the potential to enhance men's health is the school. Many adult health issues stem from the early years of life, therefore the school is an ideal setting to reinforce attitudes and behaviours for the future, whilst reaching large numbers of individuals at the same time (Smith et al 1992, Williams et al 1996).

The concept of the health-promoting school is not new; the idea was first introduced in the early 1980s and since then the concept has become more popular (Parsons et al 1996). There are three facets to the health-promoting school: the school curriculum, the school environment and community outreach (Smith et al 1992). The school curriculum includes health education which is formally incorporated into teaching and learning. Thus, topics such as substance misuse, nutrition and exercise are considered in key subject areas, such as science and physical education. The school environment includes physical aspects such as hot water and soap in toilets and washing facilities, but also a welcoming atmosphere, healthy food choices in canteens and tuck shops, non-smoking policies and a climate which fosters positive relationships between pupils and teachers. Equal opportunity policies in practice are also included. Community outreach includes involving parents and the surrounding community and environmental services to develop relationships. This might lead to reinforcement of health education through parental involvement or community service placement which may boost the pupil's self-confidence and self-awareness through developing relationships with others. Environmental project work leads to greater understanding of the wider health issues, such as housing. This aspect of the health-promoting school also provides the opportunity to develop alliances with health professionals and voluntary organizations.

The development of Healthy School Award schemes in some parts of England (Hampshire and Stockport) has facilitated progress with the health-promoting school concept. Williams et al (1996) have recently described how a nutritional focus was incorporated in an Australian school in a community with high male mortality and morbidity. Nutrition education was provided for all pupils and daily exercise was encouraged. Also, healthy food choices were provided in the canteen. Parents were included in the health activities too. Preliminary results suggest that positive changes have occurred, when compared with non-participating schools. This example demonstrates that reinforcement of health messages through organizational change and parental involvement can be successful.

SMOKING

Smoking is an important risk factor for both coronary heart disease and lung cancer in men (DoH 1992) and a great deal of effort has been focused on health promotion activities in this area over the years. Many smoking strategies have targeted the individual, using the 'helping people change' model to help people quit smoking. Reid et al (1992) cite evidence suggesting that opportunistic advice from GPs may help up to 5% of smokers to quit. However, Reid et al also believe that approaches focusing on the whole population, such as increasing tax on cigarettes, are likely to be successful too. Godfrey & Maynard (1988) suggest that increasing tax on cigarettes by 10% would reduce smoking by around 5%.

The reasons why people smoke are complex. However, cigarette advertising is likely to encourage children to commence smoking (While et al 1996). Also, evidence from Scandinavia and Japan has shown that legislation banning cigarette advertising is followed by a reduction in smoking (Economics & Operations Research Division 1992). Australian evidence from Powles & Gifford (1992) has shown that banning advertising and increasing taxes on tobacco can be useful together. The extra revenue generated from the tax increases was utilized to fund sporting and health promotion initiatives and research. Consequently, smoking statistics fell by around 10% in Australian men (around twice the reduction in British men).

It is apparent, therefore, that individual approaches to reducing smoking are not enough on their own and need to be supplemented by those that affect large numbers of people. At the same time, many individuals must work together to achieve these. Thus, smoking provides another example of how healthy public policies may promote health to men.

USE OF THE MEDIA

It seems sensible to briefly consider the use of leaflets, which are used extensively as a means of promoting health to men in primary health care and the workplace. Many feel that these emphasize the victim-blaming approach of health education. Murphy & Smith's (1993) survey demonstrated that leaflets were often given out to reinforce verbal advice or left in public places for people to access at their leisure. Interestingly, though, the professionals in the study expressed concern about the value of leaflets and their mode of use. They considered verbal back-up to be essential when handing out leaflets and few felt that leaving leaflets in public places was, in fact, useful, despite continuing to do this. More importantly, there is little quality control of leaflets and their content. Ormrod & Robinson (1994) agree that leaflets are potentially an inexpensive means of providing information, but only if the individual can acquire and understand it. Their readability measurements of five common leaflets randomly selected demonstrated that four out of the five were 'fairly difficult' to comprehend. Macleod (1997) has recently suggested that evidence from the Basic Skills Agency hints that one in six adults cannot read well enough to get by.

It follows, then, that careful planning of leaflets, coupled with evaluation of their effectiveness, is necessary to ensure that they are helpful and that men can make an informed choice regarding their health behaviour. Rosser (1996) has described how leaflets for pregnant women have been produced by asking them about their needs and carefully planning the content of these, based on research and focus groups from the target population. Campbell & Edgar (1993) also found that leaflets were predominantly aimed at adults and therefore were not suitable for use during their teenage screening sessions. However, they successfully produced a leaflet based on liaison and consultation with teenagers.

Finally, the use of the wider media may be a valuable vehicle for reaching some groups of men. Baker (1997) suggests that magazines for men have the potential to promote health. He states that 1 million magazines are now sold annually but that these are predominantly bought by men with higher incomes. Nevertheless, Baker proposes that health promoters should liaise with editors to develop articles which convey healthy messages. This may involve approaching health education from a new perspective, as Baker highlights that men are more likely to read articles which have a practical emphasis. In order to promote interest and attention, Baker proposes, for example, that safer sex is approached via an article considering lubricants and condoms, rather than discussing behaviour which might be unsafe.

CONCLUSION

This chapter has considered health promotion initiatives from a range of activities within the health promotion umbrella. Those aimed at the individual (clinics, screening and leaflets) have been discussed, along with those focusing on larger groups (community development, organizational change and health public policy). However, if men's health is to improve, it is important that health promotion activities specifically targeting men should be considered seriously. These initiatives, though, must be based on men's own expectations, beliefs and experiences of health, as Watson (1993) suggests that previously, health professionals have used their own perspective, thus minimizing effectiveness. Although it is acknowledged that this chapter does not address all the health needs of men (for example, older men are not included), this summary provides a helpful checklist of points to consider.

- Healthy public policy initiatives should be considered in order to reach more of the population.
- All practice must be evaluated from all perspectives and results disseminated. However, as Oakley et al (1995) warn, the quality of research methodology must also be carefully reviewed in order to assess the value of a practice.
- Settings should be considered in which to develop strategies.
- Community development initiatives should be flexible and local. Advertising should bear in mind the factors which will attract the target group.
- Continuity of carer should be facilitated in all developments if appropriate.
- When developing drop-in centres, local men should be involved.
- Men should be asked what their perceived needs are, although being aware of Dines et al's (1996) suggestion that young men do not always know what they need. They believe that health needs based on demographic data should also be considered.
- An informal approach (using humour if appropriate) should be fostered, especially in 'embarrassing' situations.
- Liaison between men (consumers), voluntary groups, managers, employers, planners and the media should be encouraged.
- Individual approaches may need to be reinforced by population approaches for some risk factors.

REFERENCES

Aggleton P, Homans H 1987 Education about AIDS. National Health Service Authority, Bristol
Agnew T 1996 Health video leaves teens red-faced. Nursing Times 92 (1): 8
Baker P 1996 Men only: is there a role for the well man clinic? Healthlines December 1996/January 1997: 17–19
Baker P 1997 Shelf-life. Healthlines February 1997: 10–11
Bridgwood A, Malborn G, Lader D, Matheson J 1996 Health in England 1995. What people know, what people think, what people do. HMSO, London
Bright J S 1997 Health promotion in clinical practice. Baillière Tindall, London
Brown B, Lunt F 1992 Evaluating a 'well man' clinic. Health Visitor 65 (1): 12–14

Buetow S 1996 Testicular cancer: to screen or not to screen? Journal of Medical Screening 3: 3–6

Campbell A, Edgar S 1993 Teenage screening in a general practice setting. Health Visitor 66 (10): 365–366

Cancer Research Campaign 1991 Testicular cancer. Cancer Research Campaign, London

Carroll-Williams B, Allen J 1984 Running a well-man clinic. Nursing Times 80 (6): 34–35

Chooramun R, Phee D 1997 Targeting the mental health of the nation. In: Bright J S (ed) 1997 Health promotion in clinical practice. Baillière Tindall, London

Cook R 1995 Teaching and promoting testicular self-examination. Nursing Standard 9 (51): 38–41

Davidson N 1996 Oh boys! Sex education and young men. Health Education 3: 20–23

Daykin N, Cockshoot Z 1996 Workplace health promotion and low paid employment. UWE and Avon Health, Bristol

Delaney F 1996 Theoretical issues in intersectoral collaboration. In: Scriven A, Orme J (eds) 1996 Health promotion. Professional perspectives. Macmillan Press, Basingstoke

Denny E, Jacob F 1990 Defining health promotion. Senior Nurse 10 (10): 7–9

Dines T, Cornish R, Weston R 1996 Health education needs of young men. Health Education 2: 13–18

DoH 1992 The health of the nation. HMSO, London

DoH 1993 On the state of the public health. HMSO, London

Downie R S, Fyfe C, Tannahill A 1990 Health promotion. Models and values. Oxford University Press, Oxford

Economics and Operation Research Division 1992 Effect of tobacco advertising on tobacco consumption: a discussion document reviewing the evidence. Department of Health, London

Egger G, Spark R, Lawson J 1990 Health promotion strategies and methods. McGraw-Hill, New York

Ewles L 1993 Paddling upstream for 50 years: the role of health education officers. Health Education Journal 52 (3): 172–181

Ewles L, Simnett I 1992 Promoting health. A practical guide, 2nd edn. Scutari Press, London

Family Heart Study Group 1994 Randomised controlled trial evaluating cardiovascular screening and intervention in general practice: principal results of British Family Heart Study. British Medical Journal 308: 313–320

Fareed A 1994 Equal rights for men. Nursing Times 90 (5): 26–29

Francome C, Marks D 1996 Improving the health of the nation. Middlesex University Press, London

Gerrard G E, Jones W G, Foster H 1996 TSE does not promote anxiety. Nursing Times 92 (40): 27

Godfrey C, Maynard A 1988 Economic aspects of tobacco use and taxation policy. British Medical Journal 297: 339–343

Goldbloom R B 1985 Self-examination by adolescents. Pediatrics 76(1): 126–128

Griffiths S 1996 Men's health. British Medical Journal 312: 69–70

Health Education Authority 1996 Promoting sexual health services to young people. Guidelines for purchasers and providers. Health Education Authority, London

Imperial Cancer Research Fund 1995 A whole new ball game. How to check for testicular cancer. Department of Health, London

Imperial Cancer Research Fund OXCHECK Study Group 1994 Effectiveness of health checks conducted by nurses in primary care: results of the OXCHECK Study after one year. British Medical Journal 308: 308–312

Johnson J V, Stewart W, Hall E M, Fredland P, Theorell T 1996 Long-term psychosocial work environment and cardiovascular mortality among Swedish men. American Journal of Public Health 86 (3): 324–331

Kawachi I, Colditz G A, Ascherio A et al 1996 A prospective study of social networks in relation to total mortality and cardiovascular disease in men in the USA. Journal of Epidemiology and Community Health 50: 245–251

Koshti-Richman A 1996 The role of nurses in promoting testicular self-examination. Nursing Times 92 (33): 40–41

Law M R, Wald N J, Thompson S G 1994 By how much and how quickly does reduction in serum cholesterol concentration lower risk of ischaemic heart disease? British Medical Journal 308: 367–371

Macleod D 1997 Study shows half of adults illiterate. Guardian 9th January: 6

McMillan I 1995 The life of Riley. Nursing Times 29 (48): 27–28

Morris J 1996a Should testicular cancer be recommended? Journal of Medical Screening 3: 2

Morris J 1996b The case against TSE. Nursing Times 92 (33): 41

Murphy S, Smith C 1993 Crutches, confetti or useful tools? Professionals' views on and use of health education leaflets. Health Education Research 8 (2): 205–215

Naidoo J, Wills J 1994 Health promotion. Foundations for practice. Baillière Tindall, London

Oakley A, Fullerton D, Holland J et al 1995 Sexual health education interventions for young people: a methodological review. British Medical Journal 310: 158–162

Orme J, Wright C 1996 Health promotion in primary care. In: Scriven A, Orme J (eds) 1996 Health promotion. Professional perspectives. Macmillan Press, Basingstoke

Ormrod J, Robinson M 1994 How readable are health education leaflets? Health Visitor 67 (12): 424–425

Parsons C, Stears D, Thomas C 1996 The health promoting school in Europe: conceptualising and evaluating the change. Health Education Journal 33: 311–321

Paxton S J, Sculthorpe A, Gibbons K 1994 Concepts of health in Australian men: a qualitative study. Health Education Journal 53: 430–438

Pike S 1995 What is health promotion? In: Pike S, Forster D (eds) 1995 Health promotion for all. Churchill Livingstone, Edinburgh

Powles J W, Gifford S 1992 Health of nations: lessons from Victoria, Australia. British Medical Journal 306: 125–127

Prener A, Engholm G, Jensen O M 1995 Genital anomalies and risk for testicular cancer in Danish men. Epidemiology 7 (1): 14–19

Ralph L, Seaman C E A, Woods M 1996 Male attitudes towards healthy eating. British Food Journal 98 (1): 4–6

Rees C, Jones M, Scott T 1995 Exploring men's health in a men-only group. Nursing Standard 9 (43): 38–40

Reid D J, Killoran A J, McNeill A D, Chambers J S 1992 Choosing the most effective health promotion options for reducing a nation's smoking prevalence. Tobacco Control 1: 185–197

Rissel C 1994 Empowerment: the holy grail of health promotion? Health Promotion International 9 (1): 39–47

Robertson S 1995 Men's health promotion in the UK: a hidden problem. British Journal of Nursing 4 (7): 382–401

Rosella J D 1994 Testicular cancer health education: an integrative review. Journal of Advanced Nursing 20: 666–671

Rosser J 1996 How would you like us to monitor your baby? British Journal of Midwifery 4 (1): 45–49

Rowe E 1994 A sexual health service for male sex-industry workers. Nursing Times 90 (27): 42–43

Sadler C 1985 DIY male maintenance. Nursing Mirror 12 (160): 16–18

Schaufele B 1988 Teaching testicular self-examination. Professional Nurse 3 (10): 409–411

Seedhouse D 1986 Health. The foundations for achievement. John Wiley, Chichester

Simnett I 1995 Managing health promotion. John Wiley, Chichester

Sorensen G, Thompson B, Glanz K et al 1996 Work site-based cancer prevention: primary results from the Working Well Trial. American Journal of Public Health 86 (7): 939–947

Smith C, Roberts C, Nutbeam D, MacDonald G 1992 The health promoting school: progress and future challenges in Welsh secondary schools. Health Promotion International 7 (3): 171–179

Stanford J 1987 Testicular self-examination: teaching, learning and practice by nurses. Journal of Advanced Nursing 12: 13–19

Summers E 1995 Vital signs. Nursing Times 91 (25): 46–47

Tones K, Tilford S 1994 Health education. Effectiveness, efficiency and equity. Chapman and Hall, London

Tugwell M 1996 Testicular self-examination. Primary Health Care 6 (5): 18–21

Turner D 1995 Testicular cancer and the value of self-examination. Nursing Times 91 (1): 30–31

United Kingdom Testicular Cancer Study Group 1994 Aetiology of testicular cancer: association with congenital abnormalities, age at puberty, infertility, and exercise. British Medical Journal 308: 1393–1398

Watson J M 1993 Male body image and health beliefs: a qualitative study and implications for health promotion practice. Health Education Journal 52 (4): 246–252

While D, Kelly S, Huang W, Charlton A 1996 Cigarette advertising and onset of smoking in children: questionnaire survey. British Medical Journal 313: 398–399

Williams E C, Kirkman R J E, Elstein M 1994 Profile of young people's advice clinic in reproductive health, 1988–93. British Medical Journal 309: 786–788

Williams P, Weston R, McWhirter J et al 1996 Health promoting schools: lessons from working intersectorally with primary schools in Australia. Health Education Journal 55: 300–310

Workplace Task Force 1994 The health of the nation: Workplace Task Force Report. Department of Health, London

WHO 1958 Constitution of the WHO. In: The first ten years of the WHO. World Health Organization, Geneva

WHO 1986 Ottawa charter for health promotion: an international conference on health promotion November 17–21. World Health Organization, Copenhagen

FURTHER READING

Health

Downie R S, Fyfe C, Tannahill A 1990 Health promotion. Models and values. Oxford University Press, Oxford

Naidoo J, Wills J 1994 Health promotion. Foundations for practice. Baillière Tindall, London

Health promotion

Ewles L, Simnett I 1992 Promoting health. A practical guide, 2nd edn. Scutari Press, London

Naidoo J, Wills J 1994 Health promotion. Foundations for practice. Baillière Tindall, London

Pike S 1995 What is health promotion? In: Pike S, Forster D (eds) Health promotion for all. Churchill Livingstone, Edinburgh

Scriven A, Orme J (eds) 1996 Health promotion. Professional perspectives. Macmillan Press, Basingstoke

Tones K, Tilford S 1994 Health education. Effectiveness, efficiency and equity. Chapman and Hall, London

Appendix: Useful addresses

Working with Men
320 Commercial Way
London SE15 1QN

Families Need Fathers
134 Curtain Road
London EC2A 3AR

Nottingham Men's Health Forum
Linden House
201 Beechdale Road
Aspley
Notts NG8 3EY

Men's Health Advisor
Royal College of Nursing
20 Cavendish Square
London W1M 0AB

Men's Health Advisor
North Derbyshire Health Authority
Scarsdale
Newbold Road
Chesterfield S41 7PF

Men's Health Network
Wyndcliff
17 Cowersely Lane
Huddersfield HD4 5TY

Index